MASSAGE

MASSAGE

A complete step-by-step guide

Fiona Harrold

Director of The London College of Massage

Photography by
Sue Atkinson

Foreword by
Dr Patrick C. Pietroni FRCGP, MRCP, DCH

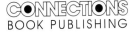

CONNECTIONS
BOOK PUBLISHING

To my darling Jamie

A CONNECTIONS EDITION
First published as *The Massage Manual* in Great Britain in 1992 by
Headline Book Publishing plc

This paperback edition published in Great Britain in 2000 by
Connections Book Publishing Limited
St Chad's House, 148 King's Cross Road
London, WC1X 9DH

British Library Cataloguing in Publication Data.
A catalogue record for this book is available from the British Library

ISBN 1-85906-047-1

1   3   5   7   9   10   8   6   4   2

Phototypeset in Garamond ITC Light and Frutiger Roman by
Bookworm Typesetting, Manchester, England
Origination by Columbia Offset, Singapore
Printed and bound in Hong Kong by Magnum Offset Printing Co. Ltd

Opposite. *Facial massage requires dexterity as this
is a small area with a great number of muscles.
A glowing complexion and younger-looking skin
can be achieved through receiving massage
here regularly*

Page 6. *Working on the front of the body
requires great sensitivity and a firm, reassuring
touch. The upper chest, in particular, can often
feel quite vulnerable.*

Contents

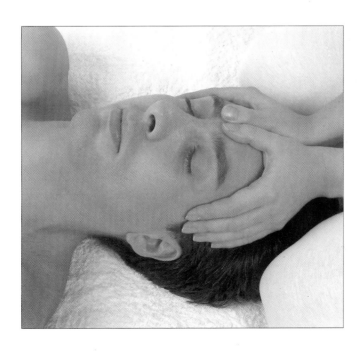

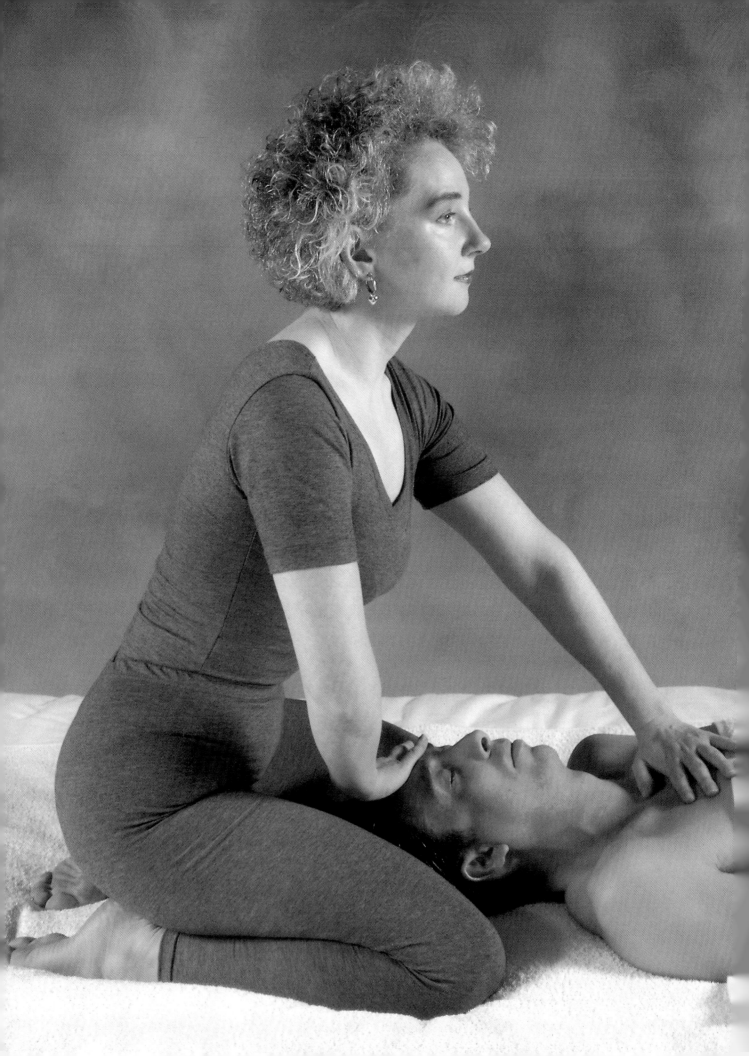

Foreword

Some years ago I started collecting old medical textbooks. I remember discovering a 'modern' textbook on cardiology dated 1890 in which there was a detailed description on the use of massage in the rehabilitation of chronic heart disease. No such chapter would be found in the intervening 100 years in a similar textbook. Future books on the subject, however, will be incomplete without one.

With the growth of interest in complementary medicine, we have begun to rediscover the importance of touch and the specific part massage can play in the treatment of many medical conditions. The discovery of vitamins, antibiotic steroids and other powerful drugs seemed to herald a new dawn in medical treatment where a 'pill for every ill' would indeed become a reality. The idea of a 'magic bullet' approach captured the imagination of the medical profession and it lost interest in the tried-and-tested natural approaches to treatment. Encouraged by the profits to be made from drugs, the pharmaceutical industry mesmerized the profession and the public alike so that a young doctor recently entering general practice after nine years of medical training was heard to say, 'If you took my prescription pad and my referral letter away, what else do I have to offer my patients?' How tragic that modern medicine could have so distanced itself from that most effective therapeutic intervention: the use of touch and the science of massage. Fortunately, in the last ten years, things have begun to change.

A recent report by the British Medical Association identified touch as one of the major reasons why people seek complementary therapies. Acupressure, shiatsu, reflexology, osteopathy and chiropractic are effective partly because the practitioners all are happy to use their hands as healing agents and not just as scientific probes. The 'laying on of hands' during spiritual healing is probably the most popular form of complementary medicine.

Massage, as Fiona Harrold suggests, is an easy, everyday skill that can be learned by almost anyone; indeed there are many cultures in which massage is taught to children in the same way as we teach our children to brush their teeth. In an eminently readable book, Fiona has provided a straightforward description of the skills of massage, which can be used on friends, lovers and oneself. In addition, the sections describing common medical conditions allow the reader to develop an understanding of how powerful and effective the use of massage can be and how it can replace the over-use of drugs on which so many doctors and patients have allowed themselves to become dependent.

Dr Patrick C. Pietroni FRCGP, MRCP, DCH
Senior Lecturer in General Practice,
St Mary's Hospital Medical School, London.
Founder-member and past Chairman of the
British Holistic Medical Association.
Principal partner in
Marylebone Health Centre, London.

Introduction

*In the final analysis, we must love in
order not to fall ill.*

SIGMUND FREUD

Massage is the oldest known healing art. It predates all orthodox medicine and all other complementary therapies. Massage is unique in being both a healing technique and an instinctive means of expression between humans and animals alike.

We all use touch without thinking of it as 'massage'. Touch is an effective means of reducing a pain, such as a headache, and giving comfort. Loving touch is best seen in the soothing caresses of a mother with her baby. For the new-born, such contact is as essential as food and warmth. Without it a baby will fail to thrive and may even die.

The benefits of quality touch are not restricted only to the very young, however. Due to its phenomenal ability to redress the ravages of stress on the body, massage has become the most popular of the complementary therapies. People everywhere are taking up massage to offer to friends and family and even to train to professional standard. From this upsurge in interest will come a wider appreciation of the unlimited, unexplored possibilities that massage has to offer us.

It is my intention that this book will provide you with a straightforward, easy-to-follow guide to getting to grips with your own healing touch. Massage is the most wonderful skill you can ever possess. The real bonus is that you will soon enjoy giving it as much as your partner likes receiving it.

The oldest healing art

In the East, massage has always been part of a valued tradition that appreciates the interrelatedness of the mind, body and spirit. It is an integral part of family life as well as a professional therapy. In the West, by contrast, medicine continues to isolate physical symptoms from the person as a whole. Recorded history shows that the Orientals were using massage at least three thousand years before the birth of Christ. The oldest existing medical text, the *Nei Ching*, acknowledges it as one of the four classical forms of medical treatments along with acupuncture, moxibustion and herbalism. In India, the *Ayurveda*, written about 1800 BC, recommends rubbing and shampooing to help the body to heal itself. The medical literature of Egyptian, Persian and Japanese physicians also makes many references to the benefits of massage.

To ancient Greek and Roman physicians, massage was one of the chief means of relieving pain. In *The Odyssey* Homer describes its restorative powers for exhausted war heroes. Hippocrates, the 'father' of medicine, believed that all physicians should be trained in massage, and in the early fifth century wrote, 'the physician must be experienced in many things but assuredly rubbing'. The Bible too, makes numerous references to the healing power of 'laying hands'.

Massage continued to thrive until the Middle Ages when the needs of the physical body and the pleasures of the flesh were suppressed and held in contempt. Christianity concentrated exclusively on the spiritual self, and created a split within the individual.

The Renaissance saw renewed interest in the body and physical health, with many prominent physicians incorporating massage into their approach. In the sixteenth century a French doctor, Ambroise Pare, brought massage to prominence and was so successful that he became the physician to four French kings; in England, Mary Queen of Scots recovered from a grave illness with the help of massage.

At the beginning of the nineteenth century

Swedish gymnast, Per Henrik Ling, synthesized his knowledge of gymnastics and philosophy with massage skills acquired in China to form Swedish Massage: a technique that remains much the same today.

The human potential and personal growth movement of the 1960s and 70s saw that massage could be a powerful agent for personal change. This attitude grew primarily out of a personal growth centre in the USA – the Esalen Institute – which sought to apply massage in a truly holistic and intuitive way. Massage was seen as a means of getting in touch with repressed emotions and memories locked within the musculature of the body. This makes perfect sense to us today, but at the time was truly innovative and heralded a return to traditional, oriental philosophies that understood the connectedness of mind, body and spirit.

The power of touch

Loving touch is vital to our emotional and physical well-being, yet it is grossly underestimated and misunderstood. As new-born babies we needed touch to survive and learned how wanted we were primarily through the quality of touch we received from our parents. We formed impressions and made decisions about ourselves, other people and life itself from this initial contact. Out of these early impressions grew our sense of worth, our self-esteem, the extent of our trust and our ease in the world. Unfortunately, child-care teaching in the West has not appreciated how crucial it is positively to affirm our offspring.

In the USA during the 1930s mothers were taught that to hold the child too much would result in a dependent child leading to a selfish, arrogant adult. Unfortunately this thinking still lingers on even today. The logic here is intrinsically flawed since needy, arrogant adults are most often those whose babyhood needs were ruthlessly denied. Babies who are not given a positive sense of their own value through loving touch grow up to have a poor self-image and very little innate self-acceptance. They are dependent on outside approval for fundamental peace of mind.

If we grow up in an emotionally cold family environment with little or no touch we feel awkward asking for or expressing affection and find it extremely difficult to form lasting, intimate relationships as adults. We may even pass this behaviour on to our own children.

It is no wonder that, as a society, we are driven to find fulfilment through possessing the right partner, house, job or car. So often happiness becomes dependent on achieving something or someone. Our culture is characterized by aggression, greed and manic competitiveness. In such an environment we feel constantly under threat, life is a perpetual struggle and we create a dog-eat-dog world.

Massage can shift this entire dynamic, and through loving touch encourage us to feel good about ourselves as we are. Through massage we can be cared for and acknowledged without having to achieve something as a condition. The better we feel about ourselves and our bodies the less dependent we will be on material gain for such fundamental security. We can be freed up to appreciate and enjoy present time and judge what we really want from the future. As long as we depend on someone or something to justify our self-worth, internal peace will ultimately elude us.

With the decline of organized religion, we no longer have the time to stand back and question the pressures and demands of our everyday life and to reflect on the future we are building. Regular massage and the meditative time out it gives brings us directly in touch with ourselves and our world. Feeling balanced and at peace with ourselves encourages us to question and justify the situations that compromise this harmony. We are more able to decide which changes, if any, we need or are willing to make to enrich and broaden our lives. Giving priority to our happiness and well-being in this way is neither selfish nor indulgent. It may well be the most significant guarantee we have of preventing illness and ensuring good health.

One of the most exciting new areas of medicine is psychoimmunology, the study of the way the mind and emotions affect the immune system. It is producing mounting evidence that stress and unhappiness prevent the immune system from fighting disease efficiently. Taking

9

care of yourself and enjoying your life can, literally, make you live longer.

Conventional medical thinking now acknowledges that stress is at the root of over 70 per cent of all illness. Professionals who take a more holistic approach would put this figure at 100 per cent, understanding that illness is merely a manifestation of a greater imbalance. Stressful events such as redundancy and bereavement frequently lead to ill-health and even death. Massage helps to reduce chronic or acute stress and so prevent the onset of illness. It also brings our attention to the fact that we are under stress, enabling us to rectify the situation before further damage is done. Once we appreciate that feeling tired and pressurized is not normal we are immediately in a position to influence our own health and vitality.

As soon as we begin to develop greater awareness of our body and its reaction to uncomfortable situations, we may notice how different feelings and thoughts result in tension in specific parts of our body. Wilhelm Reich was the founding father of modern body orientated therapy. As a pupil of Freud's, he came to realize that the body stored unresolved tensions or suppressed feelings and suggested that specific areas of 'holding' such as a tight jaw, raised shoulders, rigid pelvis or stiff neck related to specific personality types or emotions. Many of us have learned over time to keep strong emotions, such as anger, tightly locked within us. Such body 'armouring' serves to hold in the unexpressed emotion and to ward off the pain of a similar experience in the future. The price we pay is diminished vitality and a deadening of our ability to react spontaneously or to be in touch with our deeper feelings. In an attempt to protect ourselves we limit our range of experiences to ones that we hope will neither challenge nor threaten us. He also saw posture as an important map of inner tensions. If the shoulders were hunched up, it signified that the person was frightened and ready to ward off an unexpected attack. Reich's view was that physical gracefulness was an important clue to the person's emotional well-being – moving in a relaxed, easy manner indicated a healthy self. This approach has been extended by the American

therapist, Louise Hay. Through her work with clients, she has mapped out a guide to the emotion likely to be held in specific body parts.

Massage dissolves the physical tension and holding from the body, but it can also dissolve the fear and anxiety that may have created the 'armour'. Sometimes when you give a massage, a person will suddenly remember the incident that led to the tension in the first place. They may feel upset as the memory surfaces, or the emotion may simply be released and the holding dissolved effortlessly. It is only when we are at peace with ourselves that we can contribute to peace on a wider scale. It is only when we experience peace that we want to maintain it. Massage has a huge part to play in generating harmony within individuals and, as individuals, we automatically extend this well-being to others and in so doing contribute to peace and happiness on a global scale.

How does massage work?
Massage works on physical, mental and sometimes spiritual levels. It restores balance and harmony to a troubled mind and tense body, it helps us to feel better about ourselves and it leaves us with a fresh, optimistic viewpoint of life. It is the ultimate antidote to the damaging effects of chronic tension and it prevents stress from taking root in the first place. This may sound miraculous, yet experience shows that massage offers all this and more.

The human body is extraordinary in its capacity to renew and regenerate itself. Its own self-regulatory mechanism returns the body to a state of internal balance and harmony even after we stretch all its systems to cope with excessive pressures – a process known as homoeostasis.

Chronic, long-term stress inhibits this natural rebalancing. By constantly exploiting the body with unrelenting demands we deprive it of the time and energy to repair and restore itself to harmony. Massage intervenes, allowing the body to carry out its own healing by regulating the actions of the autonomic nervous system.

The nervous system divides into two processes that govern our reaction to our surroundings in complementary ways. The sympathetic system deals with the 'flight or fight' response when the

LOUISE HAY'S GUIDE TO MENTAL/EMOTIONAL CAUSES OF PHYSICAL TENSION

This is a list of the likely mental or emotional causes of some physical complaints. I have found it extremely accurate for both myself and clients, but use this only as a general guideline.

BODY PART	PROBABLE CAUSE
Head	The head represents us. When something is wrong here, it usually means we feel something is wrong with 'us'.
Neck	The neck represents flexibility in thinking. Tension here may indicate that we are being stubborn about our concept of a situation.
Throat	The throat represents our ability to speak up for ourselves and to voice our opinions or desires. Throat problems usually mean we feel unable to speak up.
Arms	The arms represent our ability to embrace the experiences of life. We store old emotions in our joints, and the elbows represent our ability to change direction.
Hands	The hands grasp, hold and clench. Grasping hands come from fear of loss or never having enough. Clenched hands cannot take in anything new.
Back	The back represents our support system. The upper back is linked to lack of emotional support. The middle back is related to guilt. The lower back is connected with material security.
Stomach	The stomach digests all the new ideas and experiences we have. When there are stomach problems, it usually means we are afraid.
Legs	Our legs carry us forward in life. Leg problems indicate a fear of moving forward or a reluctance to move in a certain direction.
Knees	The knees are concerned with flexibility. Often, when moving forward, we are fearful of bending and become inflexible. This stiffens the joints. We want to move forward but we do not want to change our ways.

body gears itself up for stress. Hormones such as adrenaline and cortisone pump into the bloodstream, the heart beats faster and the digestive functions close down. This is fine if we relax once the emergency has passed. If we carry on responding to pressure, we end up on permanent alert, wearing the body out and heading towards illness. The parasympathetic system, which reverses the 'flight or fight' reactions, is then blocked. Massage stimulates this restorative effect and induces relaxation.

We would be wise not to underestimate the importance of containing stress and replacing it with relaxation. The stress hormones released when we feel under threat can damage the body's nervous system, organs and immune system in a self-perpetuating sequence of effects. When the pituitary gland is stimulated it releases adrenaline and cortisone. If, due to unrelieved stress, cortisone continues unchecked, it suppresses the immune system, leaving the body defenceless against viruses.

Relaxation also works on the mind. In the course of our day, when we are awake, thinking, concentrating, our brain waves resonate on the 'Beta' frequency. The more anxious or angry we become, the higher we go into Beta and if we stay there for too long, we not only undermine our immune system, but become fatigued and accident-prone. Deep relaxation takes us into the much slower 'Alpha' frequency – a meditative, trance-like state that recharges us even more than sleep. Research has shown that regular meditative rest such as massage can increase immunity, improving white-cell response to stress. Massage is probably the easiest way of inducing such rest, as a chronically stressed individual may find it difficult to relax alone.

Deep relaxation is also intensely pleasurable. While in this quietened state, our body produces endorphins – hormones that relieve pain and induce feelings of contentment and even euphoria. In my experience endorphins are more effective than any drug for pain relief.

Touch is a great source of pleasure in itself. The skin is covered with nerve receptors that, when stimulated, feed the brain with enjoyable sensations. Massage is powerfully therapeutic and a life-affirming route to real pleasure.

Preparation

How you prepare for a massage significantly influences how much you and your partner enjoy it. You need to create the right environment and, equally if not more importantly, to prepare yourself.

Creating the environment

One of the prime aims of your treatment is to rid your partner of physical stagnation and mental confusion. You want to leave your partner feeling clear-headed, physically relaxed and alert. The room in which you carry out the treatment needs to reflect these qualities, offering an oasis of peace and tranquillity, a clean, clear space. This helps most people to feel good the moment they enter the room.

The ideal background colour is a warm pastel apricot or pink with similar towels. Clean, thick, soft towels feel luxurious to the skin, especially when pre-warmed on a radiator. Heat is extremely important. Your partner's body temperature will drop during the massage, so heat the room up well beforehand and keep a heater accessible if you need to boost the temperature. Your partner's muscles will not relax if the air is chilly, and the effect of your massage will be completely undermined. Make sure there are no draughts, although a little fresh air is a good idea. Always place towels over any area of the body you are not working on directly, particularly areas you have just massaged, as it is important to retain the muscles' warmth. Keep a lightweight blanket available, too, should you need it – most people feel more comfortable when they are not fully exposed.

Check that you have everything you are likely to need already in the room. This will include two large towels and a blanket, oil, tissues and music. Some people like a pillow under their head when lying on their back (although you may need to remove it to work on the neck). Some also find a pillow under the knees helps to take any strain off the lower back.

Sympathetic light also contributes to setting the mood. Avoid a direct overhead light as it can be disturbing. A side light is ideal and a candle or essential oil burner makes a lovely addition. Try to light the oil burner at least 10 minutes prior to the treatment so the aroma welcomes your partner to the massage.

I believe that music can be a great contribution to a treatment, for both giver and receiver, provided that a suitable choice is made. There are lots of wonderful, relaxing tapes available which enhance the atmosphere and support your partner's relaxation. As the giver you will benefit, relaxing into the rhythm of your massage and letting go of your own thoughts and preoccupations. Try to choose a room that will not be disturbed by outside noise. Encourage your partner to relax by not engaging too much in conversation with him or her; merely reply to any questions and let your partner know you are listening, but do not initiate conversation or prolong it. Always speak softly and quietly when you do need to speak during the massage.

The routines in this book teach how to massage on the floor. This allows you to give a treatment wherever you are, without needing a table. The ideal surface on the floor is a thick futon – a soft and comfortable Japanese mattress. Otherwise, a thick duvet will be fine. Cover your surface well with towels to protect it from the oil.

Preparing yourself

Before you give a massage, by far the most important consideration is to ensure that you are free from tension and mental preoccupations. The best way to quieten and calm yourself is to put aside at least 10 minutes before the treatment to relax consciously. Simply find a quiet place to sit or lie down and play some peaceful music quietly. Bring your awareness to your breath, noticing it without trying to change it. Become aware of any tense areas in your body and think of just letting the tension go, one part at a time. Finally bring your awareness to your thoughts and let them pass by. Do not try to stop them, simply allow yourself not to hold on to any. Then enjoy how you are feeling.

Your appearance needs to be clean and tidy. Avoid wearing noisy jewellery, watches or rings and keep long hair tied back. You would be wise to put aside specific clothes for massage, as you will invariably get oil on them. Loose, comfortable cotton is best, as are short sleeves that do not have to be rolled up out of the way.

Short nails are essential – you cannot massage with long nails. Likewise, if your skin is rough it will feel abrasive to your partner. Apply hand cream regularly and use the self-massage techniques to improve the quality of your skin. Look after your hands, the tools of your trade.

Preparing your partner

Anyone who has never received a massage treatment before, will be quite unclear as to what to do and expect. You need to explain the process clearly so there is no room for confusion. The first issue is clothes and nudity. Unless you are very close friends, I suggest that you recommend they undress to underpants – as they become more familiar with receiving massage, they may come to feel happy about undressing completely. The ideal is to work on a body free of the restrictions of clothing.

Ask your partner to remove all jewellery, including earrings, and check if they are wearing contact lenses. Some people find lying down for an hour or more with lenses in is very uncomfortable and prefer to remove them.

The massage treatment

I recommend that you initiate your massage practice by mastering the neck and shoulders routine (see pages 25–39) before moving on to work directly on the skin with oil. Use this simple sequence as a starting point to gain confidence – it is wonderfully adaptable and you can carry it out almost anywhere. When you are confident in your ability to massage, you will automatically inspire people to trust in your touch, and your friends will feel less uneasy about taking off clothes to receive massage.

Expect to spend 1 to 1 ½ hours on the entire treatment. If you want to make it shorter, omit a sequence, but 'effleurage' (see pages 16 and 17)

over the area so it does not feel neglected. You can make it longer by repeating some of the movements or giving more attention to a specific area within the full routine. If you choose to include some of the additional strokes or sequences, the treatment would then also take longer than 1½ hours.

Getting started

When your partner arrives for the treatment, both you and the room need to be totally prepared. It is your role to take total responsibility for the logistics of the treatment so that your partner is not left wondering what to do next. This means that you are clear about the steps leading up to and following the massage.

Take your partner to the treatment room with an invitation to sit down for a few minutes. Here, you need to gather a little information about the general state of health and any particular ailments. There is always a possibility, however slight, that your partner has a health condition that would not be helped by massage. This type of questioning is known as taking a 'case study'. A professional treating a serious specific condition takes a very detailed and thorough case study, but the one outlined on page 14 is succinct and quite sufficient.

Once you have completed the questions, you are ready to begin. Ask your partner to undress down to underpants, or if he or she feels comfortable, undress completely. Reassure your partner that this is entirely up to him or her and, whatever the choice, you will be equally happy, but first make sure that you are happy with this. Do not encourage a partner to undress completely if you would feel uncomfortable. Be discreet and leave the room while your partner undresses, using this time to wash your hands. Before you go, explain exactly where and how to lie – your partner must be face down for you to work on the back first.

Return to the room, cover your partner's legs and buttocks with a towel, and kneel alongside the lower back. Bring your awareness to your own breath and slowly bring your hands down to make contact on the lower back. Speak quietly and instruct your partner to breathe easily and gently, and to let his or her body sink into the

13

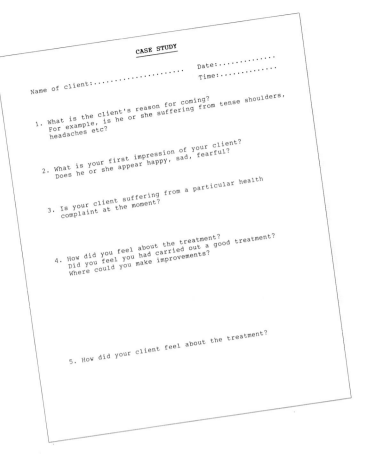

CASE STUDY

Name of client:........................ Date:..............
                                        Time:..............

1. What is the client's reason for coming?
   For example, is he or she suffering from tense shoulders,
   headaches etc?

2. What is your first impression of your client?
   Does he or she appear happy, sad, fearful?

3. Is your client suffering from a particular health
   complaint at the moment?

4. How did you feel about the treatment?
   Did you feel you had carried out a good treatment?
   Where could you make improvements?

5. How did your client feel about the treatment?

Before you start to massage someone, always make a few notes. These are useful to refer to if someone comes back to you for another treatment. Use this sample case study as a guide. Copy it so that you can keep a separate record for everyone you massage.

floor. Apply oil to your hands and begin your treatment.

Before you move on to the legs, cover the back and expose only one leg at a time for both the modesty and warmth of your partner. When it comes to turning over, hold the towel close to the body, placing it on top as your partner lies down. For extra comfort you could place a soft pillow under the head and one under the knees to take any strain off the lower back. When working on the front of the body, use towels in the same discreet manner, covering your partner completely when working on the head and face, chest and neck, and exposing only one leg at a time when working on the calves and thighs. Finally, you might like to lay a light blanket on top when you have completed the treatment, leaving your partner feeling very cared for and cocooned. Allow him or her to rest for at least 5 to 10 minutes, then complete your case study by

noting the responses made to the treatment. As a student you will need constructive feedback, so encourage your friend to be really honest and to suggest ways that you might improve.

To get the best out of this book, tackle one routine at a time. Practise it on at least three occasions until you feel comfortable with it before you move on to the next one. Whichever sequence you carry out, effleurage the rest of the body and always finish by holding the feet for at least 20 seconds. You are now well on your way to learning a wonderful skill.

Preparing the oils

We use oil in massage to provide a smooth surface for the strokes. Without it you would drag the skin and a rhythmic flowing treatment would be impossible. A good-quality organic oil such as almond, sunflower or grapeseed also nourishes the skin. To make a luxurious mixture, add 10 per cent of either jojoba, evening primrose, apricot kernel or wheatgerm oil.

You will need approximately 50 ml of vegetable oil to massage the entire body, although this will vary according to the size of your partner, the amount of body hair and the texture of his or her skin – dry skin literally drinks in the oil.

Vegetable oil is referred to as a 'carrier' or 'base' oil, when it is used as a base for essential oils, carrying them through the skin into the body. These natural herb and flower essences are therapeutic in themselves and add a further dimension of pleasure to a massage. They penetrate the skin very quickly and must never be used undiluted but always mixed into the vegetable oil. You can include them in a bath, or in an oil burner to fill a room with a particular aroma and atmosphere.

Make up enough oil for only one treatment as the oils start to lose their potency once diluted with vegetable oil. Adding 10 per cent wheatgerm oil will help to preserve the mixture from turning rancid but it does need to be refrigerated. Store all your essential oils in dark bottles as light quickly destroys their properties.

Applying the oil

The most pleasant way of applying the oil to your partner's body after making contact is to leave one hand on the body and slowly pour the oil over the back of the hand. Spread the oil onto the body with your other hand and effleurage it over the area. Otherwise, turn over one hand, keep it resting on the body and pour oil into the palm. Smooth the oil between both hands and effleurage. Use enough oil to allow you to glide smoothly over the area but not so much that you cannot knead without slipping.

At the end of the treatment, your partner may want to dry off any traces of oil. This is understandable, but point out that the essential oils are reputed to continue working, sinking into the skin for up to 12 hours after the massage.

CHOOSING ESSENTIAL OILS

Ten of the most popular and useful essential oils are listed here. Use 1 drop of essential oil to every 2 mls of vegetable oil. A full body treatment requires approximately 50 mls of vegetable oil, so you would add no more than 24 or 25 drops of essential oil. Pure rose oil is known as an 'absolute' because it is so concentrated. No more than one or two drops will have a powerful effect. All the other oils can be used individually or mixed with each other in equal proportions. A blend of three oils is ideal as they work together synergistically. Experiment to find out which blends suit you best.

OIL	PROPERTIES
Bergamot	Bergamot has the unique ability to balance, uplift and calm the mind without sedating, which makes it ideal for combating depression and anxiety. The antiseptic properties of this oil make it ideal for treating skin conditions, however, sensitizes the skin to ultra-violet light, so do not use before sunbathing.
Camomile	A distinctive fragrance that you will either love or hate, camomile is best known for its ability to calm irritation, both physical and mental. Use it on someone who is feeling very frayed and short-tempered, or on someone suffering from inflamed skin conditions such as eczema or acne. It is also useful for treating stomach cramps and pre-menstrual tension.
Frankincense	Best known for its use in religious ceremonies, frankincense has a unique woody aroma. It is particularly useful for respiratory problems and can aid relaxation. In skin care it is valued in treating wrinkles and the more mature skin.
Geranium	Best known as a hormonal-balancing oil, geranium is particularly good to use in treating pre-menstrual syndrome and the menopause. It is the perfect oil for people who experience mood swings of euphoria or depression. Men may find the aroma too floral for their taste.
Ginger	A comforting, warming oil, best used to treat dampness and water retention in the body. It brings relief to rheumatic conditions and mixes well with juniper and lavender. It is also reported to have aphrodisiac qualities. High concentrations irritate the skin, so dilute well.

OIL	PROPERTIES
Lavender	The most versatile and useful of all the oils, lavender is tremendous for relieving stress, headaches, insomnia, depression, scars and burns. It also stimulates the immune system and mixes wonderfully with many of the other oils. The aroma of lavender is appreciated by both men and women.
Marjoram	Very similar to lavender in its uses, marjoram has a much more masculine fragrance. It is a warming oil, particularly useful for muscular aches, especially exercise related, helping to increase local blood circulation. French Marjoram is useful for insomnia.
Neroli	An exquisite, delicate oil from the blossom of the orange tree, neroli is the classic stress remedy: calming, uplifting and reassuring. It is also a beneficial oil for the skin with the ability to encourage cell regeneration.
Rose	The 'queen' of essential oils, rose is an all-purpose general tonic, but particularly useful for the nervous, circulatory and respiratory systems. It is wonderful in massage after childbirth and, like neroli, it is very good for skin complaints, from wrinkles and dryness to eczema. Be sure to buy only pure rose oil. The best types are Bulgarian or Moroccan.
Rosemary	A stimulating, uplifting oil, rosemary is beneficial for all types of congestion and mental and physical sluggishness. Use for sinusitis, headaches, poor memory, migraine, coughs and flu, fluid retention, cellulite and rheumatism. It is a wonderful pick-me-up and ideal in a morning bath or before an evening out.

The Basic Strokes

Massage is an instinctive and intuitive healing art at everyone's fingertips. Over the generations, however, certain strokes and techniques have been perfected to enhance the pleasure and specific effects of a treatment. To fulfil the therapeutic potential of the massage, the strokes need to be given in a particular way and in a certain order.

A treatment always opens with 'making contact'. This is true whether the treatment is to last 15 or 90 minutes. Making contact slows you down, setting the tone of the treatment. You then move on to effleurage, which relaxes not only the area you are working on but also the entire body. This paves the way for you to work deeper with petrissage and kneading strokes, releasing layers of tension in the muscles.

Kneading opens the muscles for still deeper release with friction strokes. It is imperative to prepare the body thoroughly in this way, as failure to warm the muscles sufficiently would make the friction extremely unpleasant to re-

FLAT-HAND EFFLEURAGE
Effleurage is the simplest and most instinctive of all massage strokes, and one we all use unwittingly at some time, to ease a headache, pacify a sharp pain or ease tension. Effleurage translated from the French means 'stroking', and it is this rhythmic stroking movement that is so ideal to open a treatment, relaxing both the specific area and the whole person, while preparing the muscles for deeper work. Effleurage is used everywhere on the body although it can look quite different from one place to another. On the back, we use a flat-handed effleurage due to the wide flat surface available. The stroke here is always carried out with relaxed flat hands with the momentum on the upward stroke (*see top right*) and no pressure on the return stroke (*see bottom right*). The reason for this is physiological – to enhance the overall circulation of the blood and lymph, carrying waste products to the lymph nodes for processing and elimination.

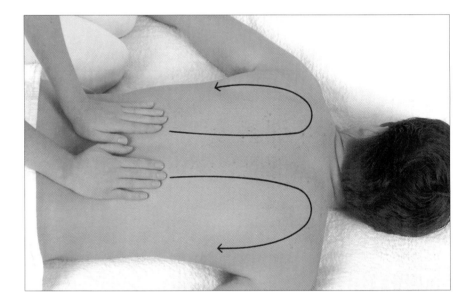

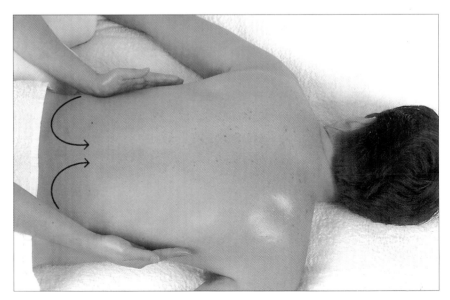

ceive. The therapeutic impact of the strokes would also be seriously undermined, reaching only the outermost layers of the muscle, and the muscles may react to the intrusion by going into spasm. Your partner would undoubtedly feel worse than before the treatment. Percussion strokes, if you are using them at all, are introduced at this stage or at least after the kneading, when the body is thoroughly warmed up.

Finally, the treatment is completed with effleurage and 'holding' the body as you did at the outset. This sequence is not only common-sense but makes for a more therapeutic treatment.

The formal structure of strokes and routine is invaluable at the beginning when you are likely to be unfamiliar with touching yourself or someone else in this close, nurturing way. It is essential to acknowledge massage as an artform with a particular discipline, and to master the fundamentals before allowing yourself too much creative freedom. There is a strong temptation to interpret the techniques in your own way – this may be fun for you, but is likely to feel unfocused and sloppy to your partner.

This chapter presents a thorough explanation of each of the main massage techniques – information that neads to be absorbed before you go on to the actual hands-on sequences. Ultimately you can only learn from having a go, but this information will nonetheless help you and increase your confidence.

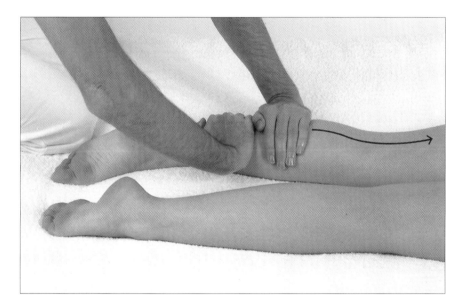

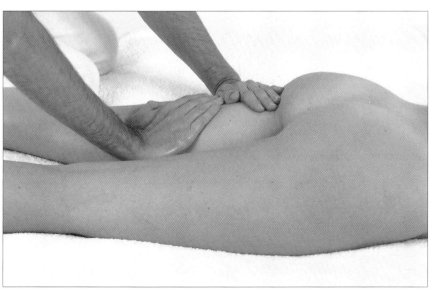

CUPPED-HAND EFFLEURAGE
Effleurage is particularly soothing on the calf muscles which are often extremely sensitive. If circulation is poor and varicose veins are in evidence, light effleurage is the only stroke you can safely use. The great value of this light effleurage is to assist the return of the lymph fluid to the large clearing ducts in the groin. A sluggish lymphatic return in this area leads to the common problems of fluid retention and cellulite in the thigh and buttock areas. Effleurage, increasing the flow upwards, directly helps the body to regulate itself. The stroke is carried out with cupped hands wrapped sideways around the leg (*see top left*). It is especially important to position the hands so your inside hand can turn discreetly on your partner's inner thigh (*see bottom left*).

17

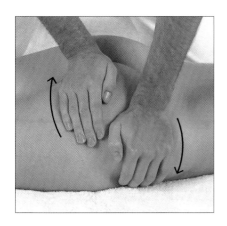

PETRISSAGE

Petrissage is the term for any stroke that squeezes the muscles, including kneading and wringing. It is unsurpassed in its ability to literally squeeze toxins and tension out of the muscles. The return of fresh blood and oxygen allows the body to regulate and renew itself once again. Petrissage is most effective when used on the shoulders, legs and buttocks. You can use both hands to squeeze into the muscle in opposite directions (*see above and right*) or squeeze with one hand and rest the other on the leg (*see below*). This stroke is most effective with quite strong pressure, but respond to the area you are working on, and the extent of your partner's tightness.

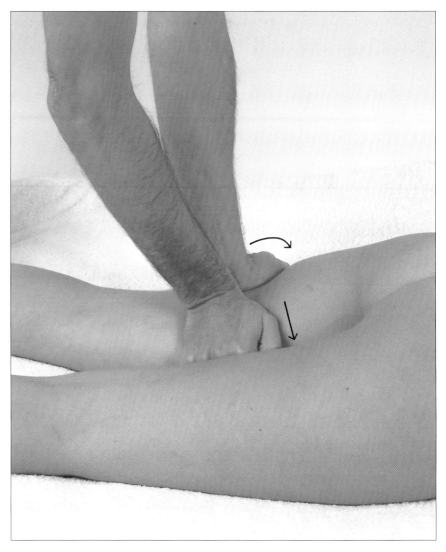

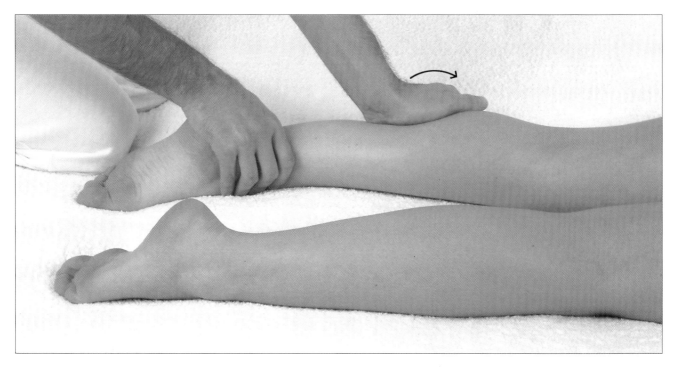

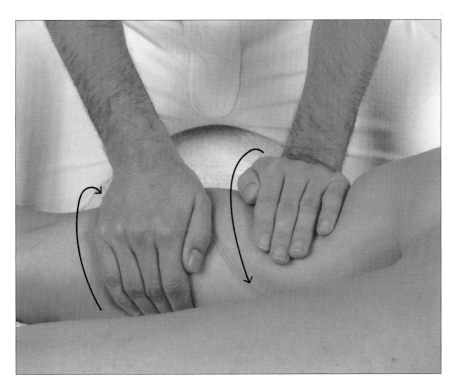

WRINGING

When performed correctly wringing literally wrings tension and trapped toxins out of the muscles. It is most effective combined with kneading on the large muscles of the calves and thighs. Wringing on the thigh is performed with the thumb close to your other fingers (*see left*). On the calf, you keep your thumbs open wide to get a very firm grip on the muscles as you wring them (*see below*).

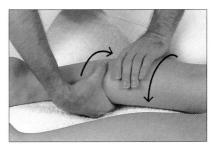

KNEADING

Kneading is the most well-known and widely used stroke of the petrissage family. It is extremely versatile, forming part of a calming, relaxing massage or contributing to an invigorating, stimulating treatment. The slower and deeper the movement, the more effective it is in squeezing tension and congestion out of the muscles. The more vigorous the movement, the more you stimulate the circulation and wake up the entire body. It is wonderful on the fleshy areas of the body like the buttocks and thighs, although it is also useful on the calves. Never knead on the legs if there are varicose veins or broken capillaries. To make the stroke effective, lean your hand firmly into the muscle before your squeeze it between your fingers and thumb (*see left*) and ensure your hands work rhythmically together, flowing towards each other. Failure to lean into the muscle means you may merely pinch the flesh.

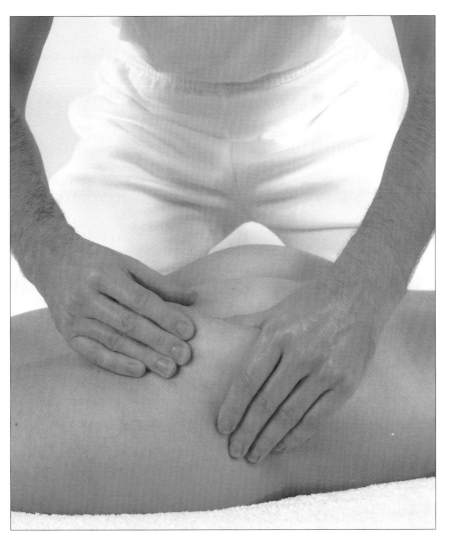

19

CIRCULAR KNUCKLING

Knuckling is universally popular. It can be used lightly on the upper chest to relax the muscles and to encourage the shoulders to release tension, or it can be worked deeply into the pectoral muscles to ease stubborn or long-standing tension. Knuckling feels good on the back of the hands and, provided the pressure is firm, can be very satisfying on the soles of the feet. You curl your hands into loose fists and, with the middle section of your fingers on the skin, rotate your fingers in a circular movement.

STRAIGHT KNUCKLING

On the thighs and buttocks you keep your knuckles flat on the skin and do not rotate your fingers. This form of knuckling reaches deep into the muscles and tissues to break up stubborn fatty deposits and prizes tension from muscles. The movement involves curling your hands into loose fists and gliding firmly up the leg with the middle section of your fingers. Always work up the leg to assist blood from the veins to return to the heart and lymph flow to the lymph nodes in the groin, but never use this stroke if varicose veins are a problem.

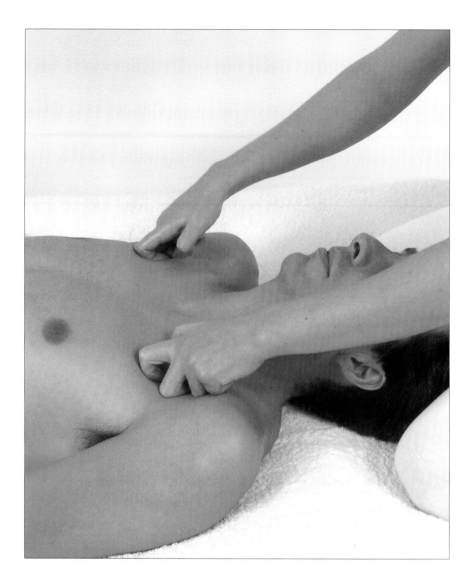

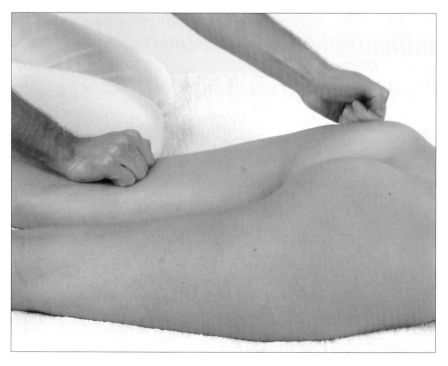

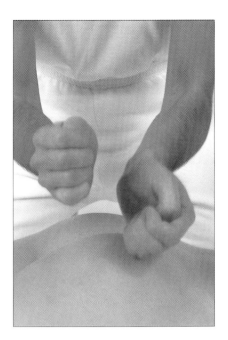

PUMMELLING

Pummelling is the simplest of the two percussive movements featured in this book (*see left*). It is a stimulating, energizing movement that disperses chronic, stubborn tension and increases the blood flow to the area, leaving it tingling with energy. Because of its stimulating power, avoid pummelling if your partner is frail, elderly or needs complete relaxation. Limit this stroke to the padded fleshy areas of the body, such as thighs and buttocks. Here, its powerful impact helps to break up fatty deposits and congestion, bringing life and lustre.

HACKING

Hacking is the most dynamic of the percussive movements (*see below*). It performs the same role as pummelling and brings the same cautions, but it takes a great deal more practice to perfect, and it is advisable to practise on your own thighs in the beginning! The two essential ingredients of the art of hacking are relaxed hands and wrists and rhythm. The edge of each hand hits the body in rapid succession with the little finger folding into your hand each time. Check that your hands do not become rigid and keep the movement slow and rhythmic.

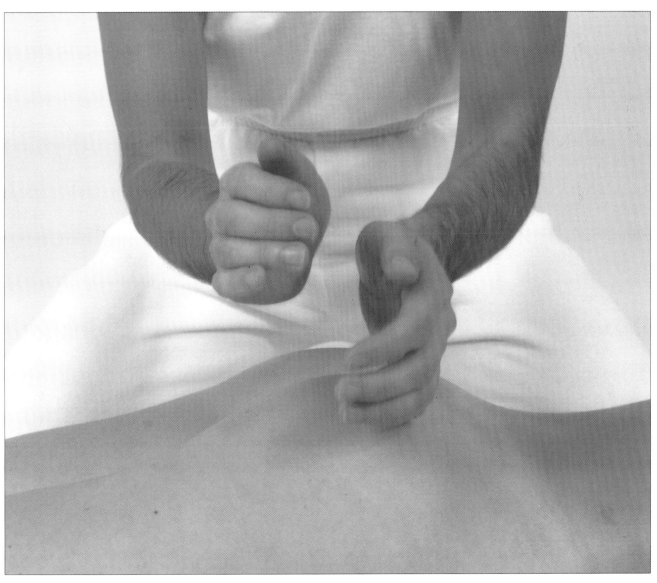

CIRCLING

Circling is a friction stroke which works deeply into the muscle through pressure and slow rotation. It works well on any area that requires very deep pressure, such as the back, the tops of the shoulders and the calves. On the spine, it serves to relax the muscles and nerves that extend out from the backbone itself. You place one hand on top of the other with the fingers relaxed but straight, lean into the muscles and slowly rotate in small circles. When circling on the knee, you use the thumbs instead of the fingers.

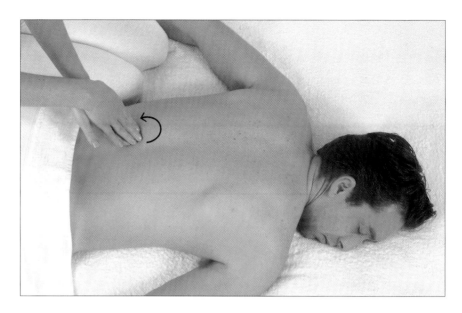

THUMB ROLLING

This stroke works to smooth out knots in the muscle fibres and to iron out uric acid deposits which collect where tension inhibits the flow of blood to the area. It is particularly useful on the upper back in the area between the spine and the shoulder-blade. Using the length of your thumbs you press into the flesh, one thumb after the other in a rhythm, leaning the whole of your body weight into your thumbs to produce a powerful movement.

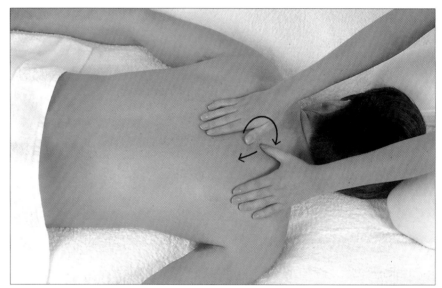

FEATHERING

Feathering should be used when completing a sequence. It is soothing, calming and heightens the sensitivity of the skin you have been working on. It can also smooth down a person's auric energy, the energy around the body, leaving a particularly relaxing and pleasant feeling. Simply stroke your fingertips lightly down your partner's back and gradually lighten your contact until your fingers are gliding slightly above the skin.

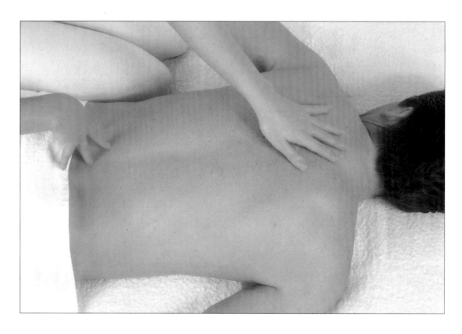

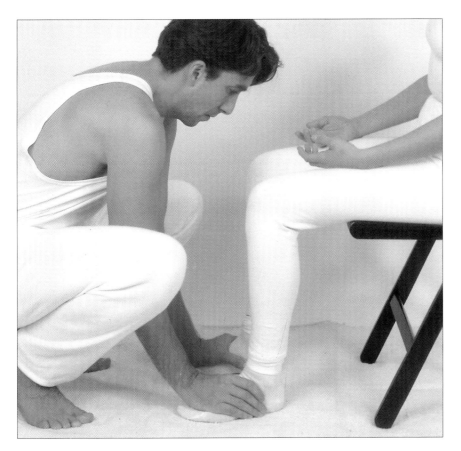

GROUNDING

Completing your treatment in a caring, sympathetic manner is very important and sets the seal on a good treatment. At the end of a massage your partner will be feeling very relaxed and possibly quite distant. It would be quite wrong and certainly counterproductive for them to get up immediately – their minds will be quiet and slow and an abrupt change of gear would probably lead to a headache. It is also very therapeutic for them to acknowledge and savour the waves of profound relaxation rippling through their mind and body. Grounding quite simply means bringing your partner's awareness back to their feet. After a treatment on the upper part of the body grounding is especially important – your partner would feel out of sync or disjointed if you failed to make contact with their feet. However you begin your massage, always complete it by holding the feet for at least 20 seconds.

Once you begin

You are now ready to begin your first massage. No doubt you are feeling excited, enthusiastic and maybe even a little apprehensive. This is perfectly understandable. Learning a new skill always makes us a little nervous. However, once you get started and begin to relax yourself, you will become so caught up with your partner and what you are doing, you will let go of any anxiety.

You will be surprised at how little you have to do for your partner to appreciate and benefit from your touch. As long as you have a clear intention of wanting to help your partner to feel good, your care will be expressed through your touch. It is more important to convey gentleness and sympathy in your touch than to master the strokes with expertise.

I have sometimes received a wonderful massage from an inexperienced but caring and dedicated student and often experienced a careless, perfunctory treatment from a professional who was bored and jaded. Simply performing the strokes correctly never adds up to a wonderful, relaxing massage. At the same time, learning to master the various movements will mean you offer the best possible treatment.

One of the best and most pleasurable ways to learn massage is by receiving it yourself. Find a good therapist and experience the many benefits of regular massage, or study this book with a friend and practise on each other. Either way, make sure you do not neglect yourself when you are giving so much to others.

Points to remember

1. The first touch is vital – be gentle.
2. Relax! You are probably doing fine.
3. Breathe and drop your shoulders.
4. Be comfortable. If you are tense yourself, you cannot give a good treatment or enjoy giving. Change your position until you are at ease.
5. Keep your hands in full contact with your partner's body, moulding them to its contours.
6. Lean your weight in to give firm pressure.
7. Encourage relaxation by not initiating conversation. Speak softly if you do need to speak.
8. Set up a rhythm. Keep your massage flowing and continuous, moving from one stroke into the next. Use effleurage to connect your movements.

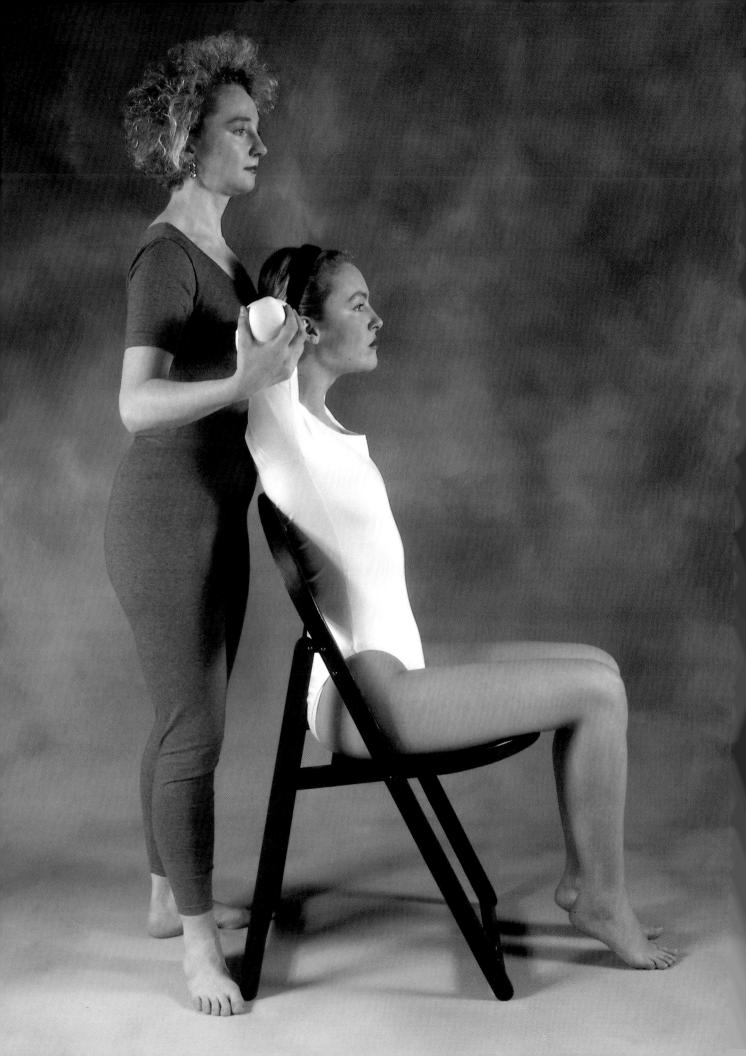

1

Neck and Shoulders Without Oil

A neck and shoulder massage is almost always welcome as it is quite rare to find someone who does not have tension in this area. Poor posture is usually the cause of this tension. Bad habits are often acquired at school: we sit in unsupportive chairs for hours every day, placing great strain on the upper back. Carrying the head way out in front of the body, which many of us do unconsciously, further tightens the muscles of the upper back and shoulders.

The human body is designed to move and inactivity consolidates posture problems. Immobilizing the body for hours every day means that we need to take special care of ourselves. A sedentary lifestyle, such as the modern office worker's, sets us up for chronic neck and shoulder pain, tension headaches and Repetitive Strain Injury (RSI). Massage is essential to release these tension patterns and give our body the opportunity to realign itself. If you are studying a postural-awareness technique such as the Alexander Technique, massage can be of great benefit.

Psychological factors influence the way in which we carry our neck and shoulders. An individual with lifelong rounded shoulders is likely to have a defensive personality, as this posture serves to protect the vulnerable chest area. Massage has the potential to smooth out fear and mistrust. A sympathetic, reassuring neck and shoulder treatment helps alleviate anxiety and instil calm.

This sequence is wonderful to carry out
on friends who are new to massage. It feels
very safe as they can remain fully
clothed throughout.

Neck and Shoulders Without Oil

The shoulders are the weakest part of the body for both men and women. Almost universally, this area is also the most tense and troublesome. This is due to both lack of use and misuse of our body in this region. The shoulder-joint in conjunction with the shoulder-blade is the most flexible of all the joints, allowing the arms tremendous range of movement. It is only by moving the arms freely through this range that the shoulder-blades and surrounding muscles are kept mobile and loose. Lack of exercise and a sedentary lifestyle mean that these activities rarely take place.

The trapezius muscle dominates this area. This is a huge muscle, which holds the shoulder-blades in place. It runs up both sides of the neck, across the top of the shoulders, reaching down to the middle of the back. If the trapezius is abnormally contracted or restricted, it will lead to discomfort in all these areas.

The upper trapezius stabilizes the head when the neck is bent forward. Witness the office worker hunched forward over a desk for hours. Contracting the muscle like this involves a great strain. This is also true when the head is permanently pushed forward due to bad posture.

The middle trapezius lies across the top of the shoulders. Here the muscle acts to brace the shoulders, holding the shoulder-blades in place. We often tense this muscle when driving. A stressful journey can result in a burning pain between the shoulders as we clench our fists on the steering wheel, pulling the shoulder-blades aggressively forward. Cold weather or emotional factors will lead us to draw the shoulders in. Tension in the muscle here will also show in hunched-up shoulders held unnaturally high.

The lower trapezius is located in the middle part of the back, passing upwards and outwards to the shoulder-blades. This section is not as relevant to the neck and shoulder region as the middle and upper trapezius.

THE NECK AND SHOULDER MUSCLES EXPLAINED

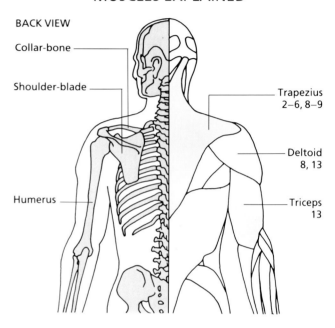

BACK VIEW

Collar-bone

Shoulder-blade

Humerus

Trapezius 2–6, 8–9

Deltoid 8, 13

Triceps 13

Numbers refer to steps in the following sequence, showing at which stage each muscle is worked upon.

The trapezius is the muscle most likely to cause neck and shoulder tension. The following sequence works primarily on this muscle, mainly where it runs along the tops of the shoulders and up the neck to the base of the skull. The deltoid, biceps and triceps muscles will be painful if Repetitive Strain Injury (RSI) is a problem. The latissimus dorsi will only be reached if you continue massaging down the back pressing thumbs either side of the spine.

Other muscles directly worked on in the following sequence are the deltoid, biceps and triceps. The deltoid wraps around the shoulder-joint, giving it its rounded appearance. The biceps covers the front of the upper arm and the triceps the back. These muscles may well ache in someone who is suffering from Repetitive Strain Injury (RSI) (*see Common Ailments, page 39*) or has over-exercised. Squeezing the upper arm is often effective in bringing relief.

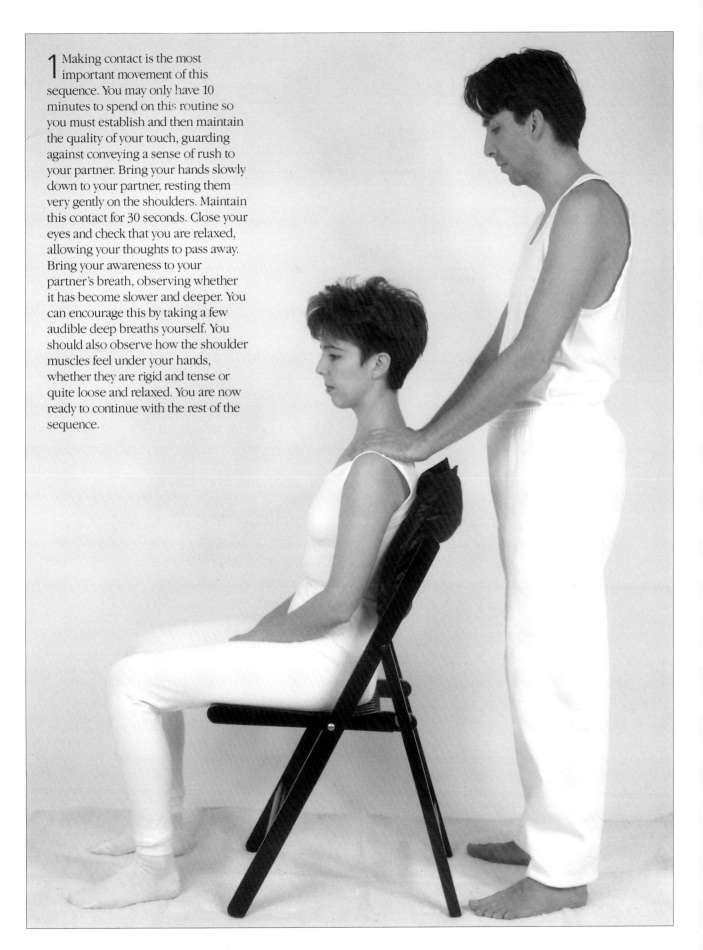

1 Making contact is the most important movement of this sequence. You may only have 10 minutes to spend on this routine so you must establish and then maintain the quality of your touch, guarding against conveying a sense of rush to your partner. Bring your hands slowly down to your partner, resting them very gently on the shoulders. Maintain this contact for 30 seconds. Close your eyes and check that you are relaxed, allowing your thoughts to pass away. Bring your awareness to your partner's breath, observing whether it has become slower and deeper. You can encourage this by taking a few audible deep breaths yourself. You should also observe how the shoulder muscles feel under your hands, whether they are rigid and tense or quite loose and relaxed. You are now ready to continue with the rest of the sequence.

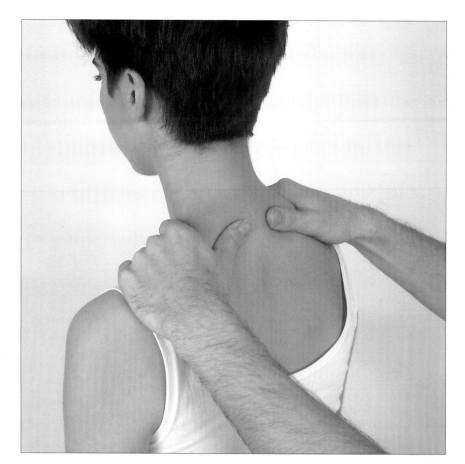

2 Begin to squeeze the shoulder muscles slowly and gently between the heel of your hand and your fingers. Your thumbs do not come into this movement at all. Increase the depth and pressure of the squeeze very gradually. Work from the inside of the muscle, nearest the neck, across the shoulder out towards the arms. This is a very simple movement, but one that feels very soothing to your partner and opens up the muscle for the next stroke.

3 Step back from your partner. Place one foot in front of the other and bend your front knee. Lean your body weight into your thumbs. Press your thumbs into the shoulder muscles and rotate slowly. Do not rotate your thumbs until you have fully conveyed your body weight into them or this stroke will be ineffectual and feel quite irritating. It is also important to rotate the thumbs very slowly for a thorough and relaxing movement. Work fully on the muscles, covering the entire breadth of the shoulders. When you are confident with the entire neck and shoulder sequence, you may insert additional step 3a here (*see page 37*).

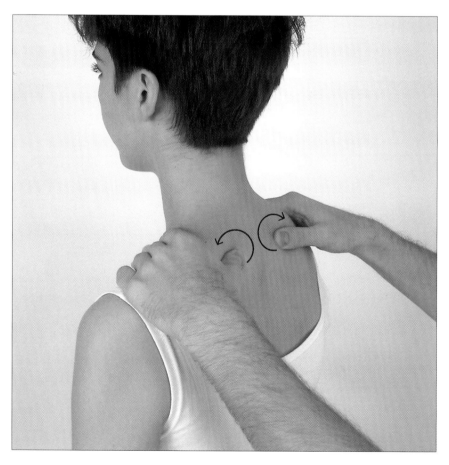

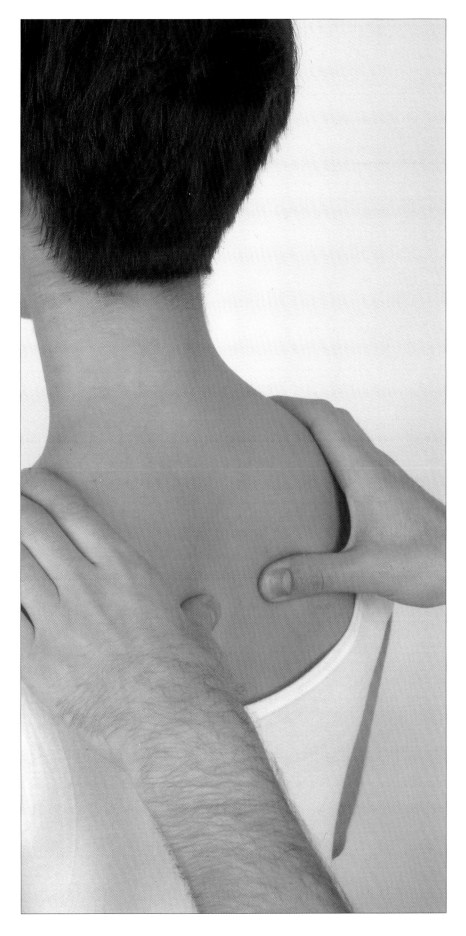

4 Place your fingers firmly over the top of the shoulders to anchor your hands. Position the thumbs at the top of the back, either side of the spine. Drop your weight into your thumbs as you lean forward (*see left*). Press down the spine in this way until you are half-way down the back or reach the chair. As with step 3, it is imperative that you co-ordinate leaning your body weight and pressing your thumbs. Without this weight your thumbs will merely be pushing into the body, which will feel uncomfortable and even invasive. Check with your partner to find out how much pressure is comfortable.

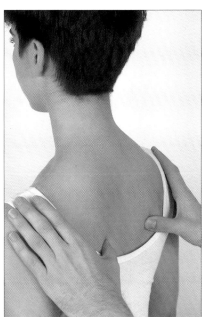

5 Bring your hands to rest firmly on the shoulder-blades. Lean the thumbs into the back at the top of the shoulder-blades (*see above*). Use your body weight as in steps 3 and 4. Work slowly and thoroughly around the shoulder-blades to the bottom then back up and around the blades to the top until they have been completely treated. Keep the rest of your hands in firm contact with the body throughout this movement, moving only to facilitate the working of the thumbs.

6 Move to your partner's side, keeping a hand on her back meanwhile to maintain contact. Bring your other hand onto her forehead, making sure her hair is over your hand. Move your hand from the back up onto the neck (*see main picture*). Encourage your partner to relax her neck and head by letting her head rest on your hand. Begin to squeeze the neck muscles upwards between your fingers and thumb in a circular motion. Work thoroughly up the neck to the base of the skull. Be extremely careful not to include the throat in this movement. Make the position of your hand appropriate to the size of the neck. If your hand is quite large in comparison to the neck, then the squeezing should be done with the fingertips and thumb. With smaller hands and a larger neck, the full length of the fingers should be used. When you have worked thoroughly on one side begin the next stroke before moving to the other side. Continue to support your partner's head with your hand.

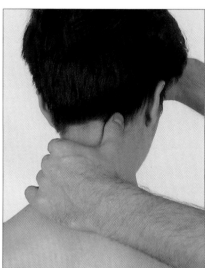

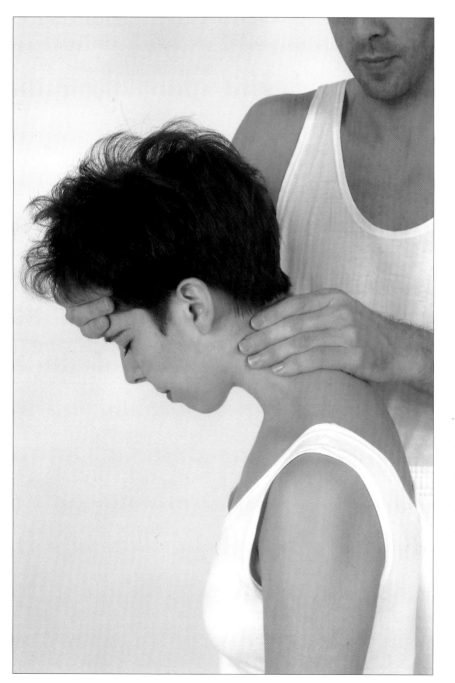

7 Lean your thumb up and into the ridge along the base of the skull near the ear (*see above*). Hold this pressure for at least 10 seconds. Use the ball of your thumb to press upwards and then inwards, rotating very slowly. Work towards the centre of the ridge, but only as far as your thumb will comfortably reach. When you have completed one side, move to the other to carry out steps 6 and 7. When you are confident with the entire neck and shoulder sequence, you may insert additional steps 7a, b and c here (*see pages 38–39*).

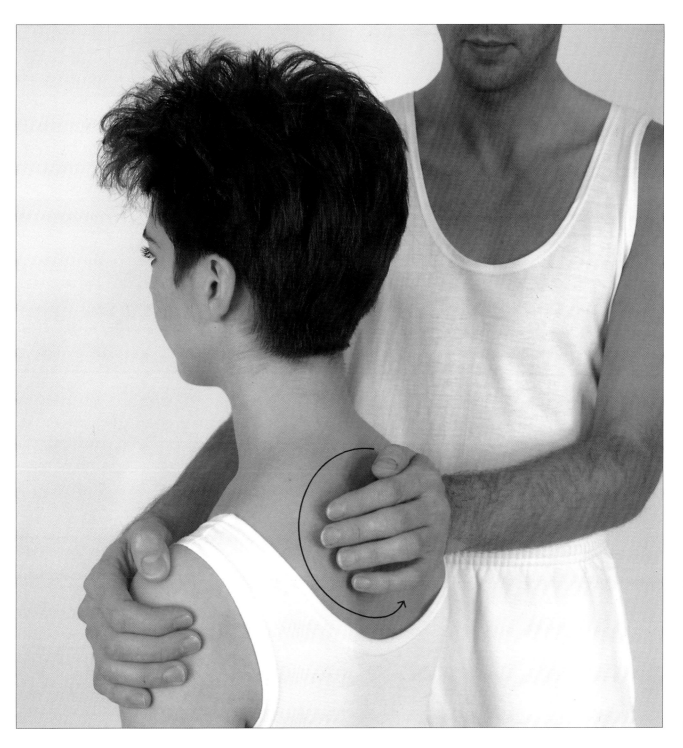

8 Still standing by your partner's side, stabilize her body by bringing one hand around to the front and holding the shoulder. Lean forward slightly to apply pressure. Rotate the heel of your hand all over the upper back. Pay particular attention to the area around the shoulder-blades. Begin slowly and increase to a vigorous pace, maintaining precise movements.

9 Move behind your partner again. Bend your knees slightly and rest your forearms on your partner's shoulders. Concentrate on the muscles closest to the ears first of all, remaining there for at least 10 seconds. Then move towards the arms, being careful not to rest on bone itself. Do not press into the shoulders but transfer some of your weight to them. Use the sides of your forearm, not the flat inner part.

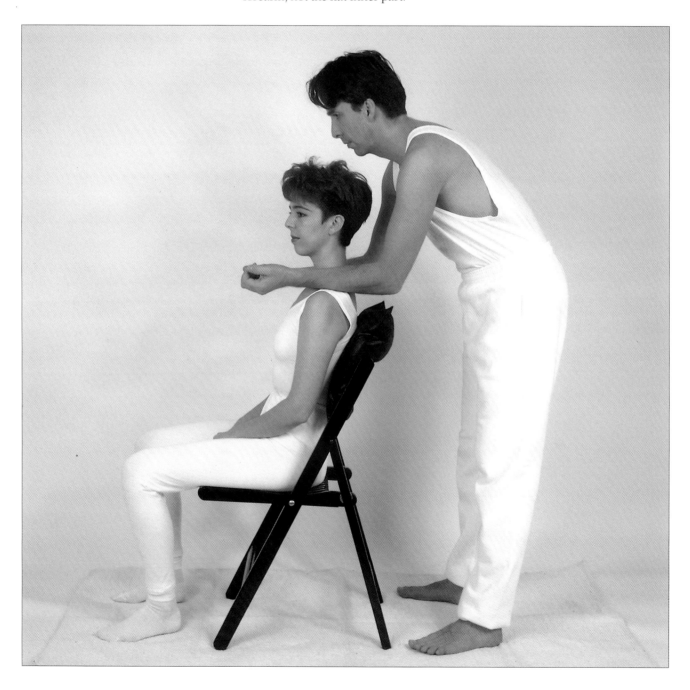

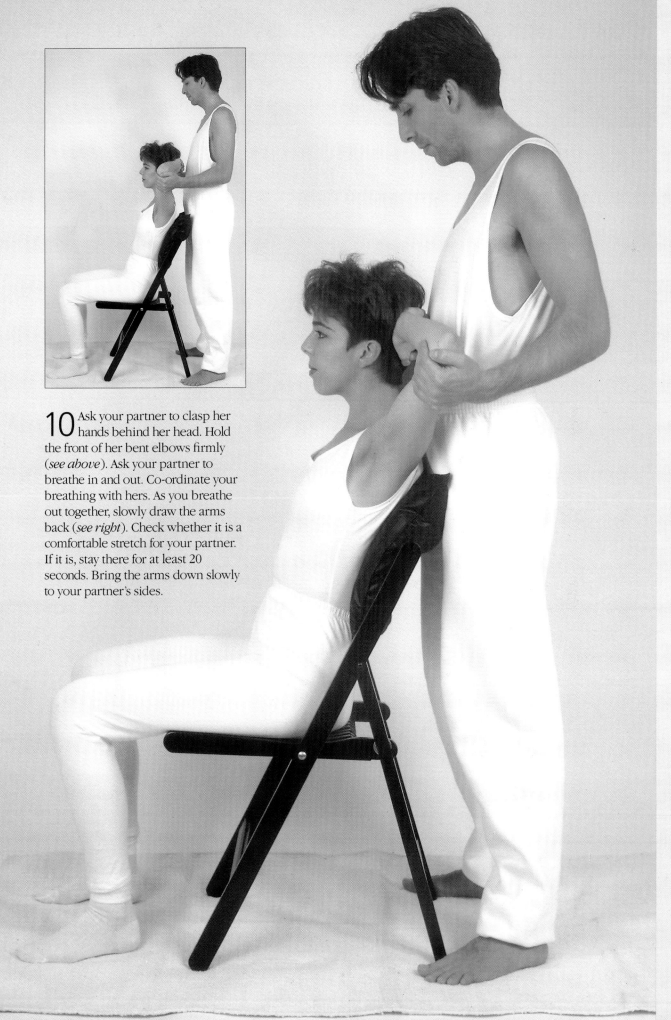

10 Ask your partner to clasp her hands behind her head. Hold the front of her bent elbows firmly (*see above*). Ask your partner to breathe in and out. Co-ordinate your breathing with hers. As you breathe out together, slowly draw the arms back (*see right*). Check whether it is a comfortable stretch for your partner. If it is, stay there for at least 20 seconds. Bring the arms down slowly to your partner's sides.

11 Place one hand on the forehead. Draw the hand back towards you over the head, stroking slowly. As soon as you reach the hair, bring the other hand onto the forehead to follow your first hand. Draw the hands simultaneously over the hair and down the back as far as you can reach. Keep your touch light. Repeat four to five times, making the stroke lighter each time so that you are barely touching your partner by the final stroke.

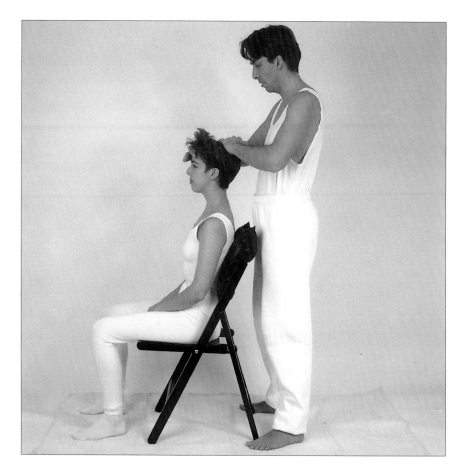

12 Begin with your hands held over the top of the head. Slowly draw the hands very lightly down onto the head. Continue down the sides of the head onto the shoulders and down the arms to the elbows. Close your eyes and repeat the movement in exactly the same way, letting your contact become lighter and lighter. You will be surprised how pleasant your partner will find the sensation. Even though you are barely touching the skin, she will still feel that you are in touch with her.

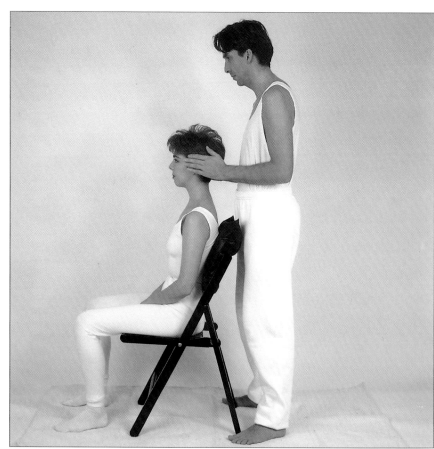

13 Bring your hands to the top of the arms, just below the shoulder-joint. Lean your body slightly and squeeze the arms gently. Do this movement very slowly and thoroughly and then slide the hands down to the next section of the arms. Be very methodical in your approach. This stroke is best if carried out gently but quite firmly, as it is not meant to be uncomfortable. It should feel very pleasant and will affect the entire upper-body region. Suggest that your partner closes her eyes if she has not done so already. Work as far as the elbows. Repeat.

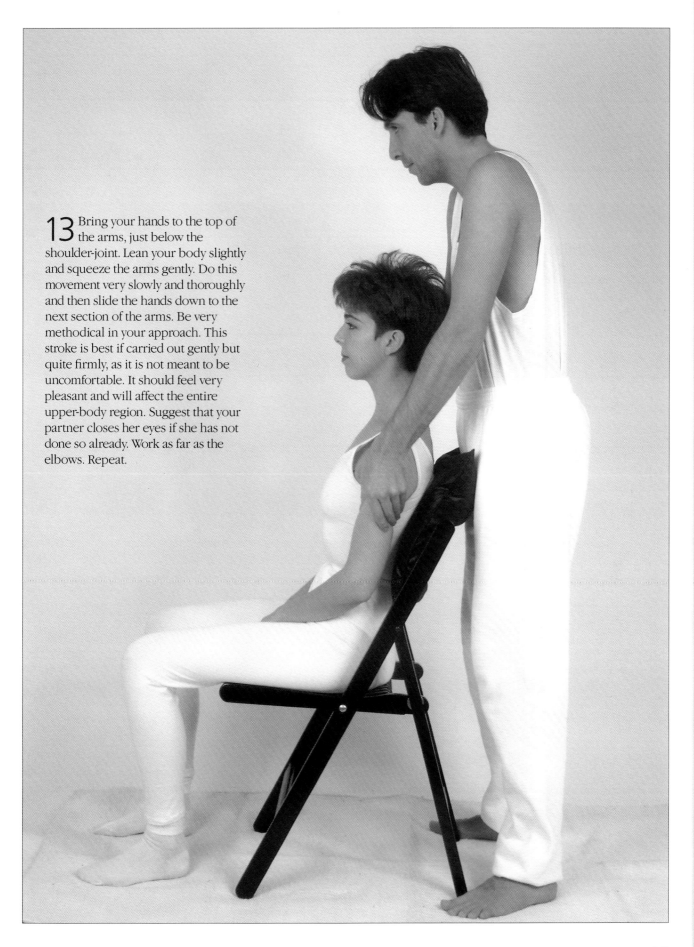

14 Come round to the front of your partner's body. Bring your hands to the knees (*see right*) and glide them slowly down the legs to the ankles (*see below*). Squeeze the legs gently as you do so. Hold the feet for at least 10 seconds. This is a very important 'grounding' or 'earthing' stroke. It brings your partner's attention away from the upper body to her contact with the ground. Without it your partner may feel a little light-headed. Encourage her to stay still and rest for a few minutes.

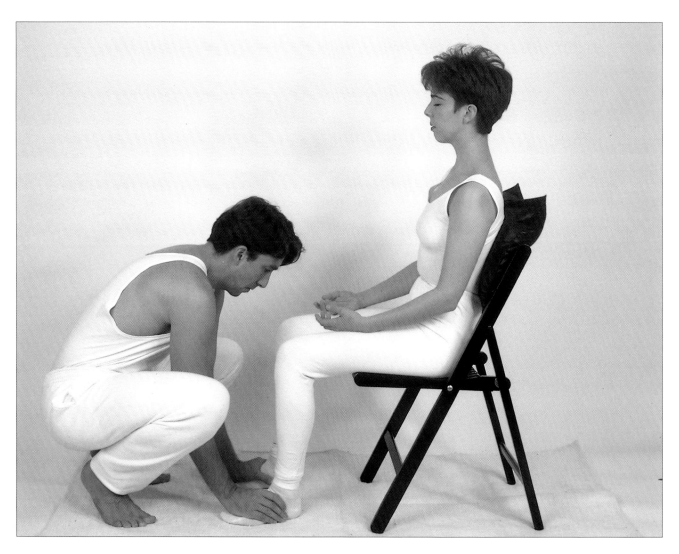

Additional Steps

Once you are confident with the previous neck and shoulder routine, you might like to try a few additional steps. The following, optional movements can easily be incorporated into the routine but, they should not be added on at the end. The captions explaining the additional steps tell you at what stage in the routine each one should be introduced. The strokes on pages 38 and 39 focus on the neck, base of skull and head. These very simple movements concentrate on releasing neck tension. They are all useful for helping to reduce a headache, but rotating the fingers on the base of the skull and the scalp is of the greatest benefit.

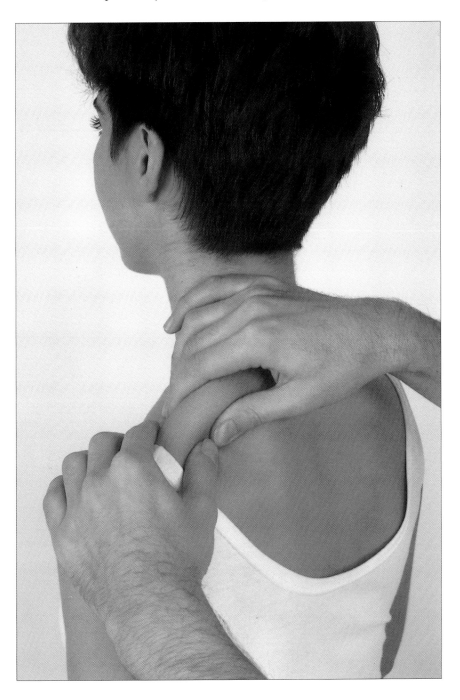

3a This stroke can be carried out after step 3, rotating the thumbs into the shoulders (*see page 28*). Bring both hands to one shoulder at a time. Anchor your thumbs by wrapping the fingers firmly onto the front of the shoulders. Push the thumbs into the muscle and squeeze using fingers and thumbs together. Push the thumbs off the muscle and move to a different part. Gradually increase the pressure of your thumbs so that they affect deeper layers of muscles. Work over the muscle thoroughly and then move hands to the other shoulder.

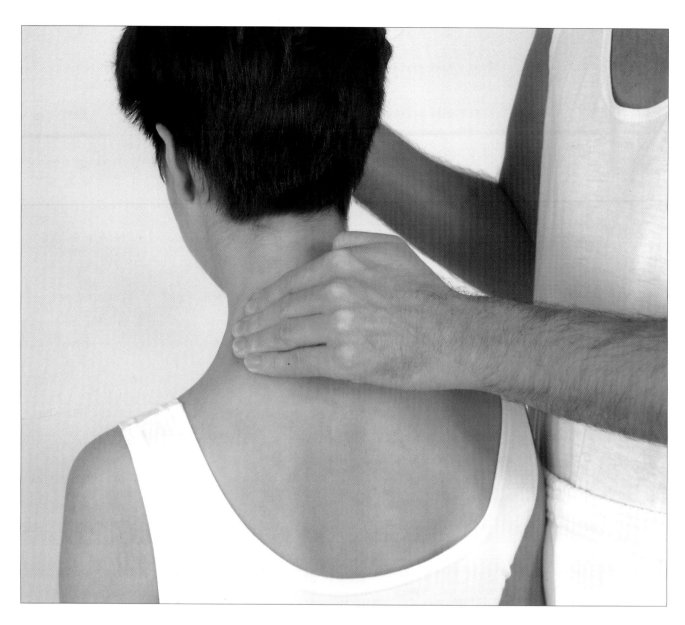

Use the following three strokes after step 7 when you have softened the neck muscles with kneading (*see page 30*).

7a Place your fingers on the side of the neck furthest away (*see above*). Press the balls of your fingers into the muscles and rotate them very slowly. Make sure that you are rotating into the muscles, not just over the skin. Work up the neck to the base of the skull. Stay on this side for the next two strokes.

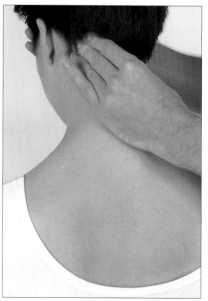

7b Press the fingers inwards and upwards along the base of the skull (*see left*). Allow your partner's head to drop forward slightly, if it has not already done so, to expose the base of the skull. Be careful not to press your hand into the forehead but to 'catch' the head as it relaxes forward. Keep your finger movements small, slow and precise. This area is often tender with a great deal of trapped tension. Find out from your partner how much pressure is acceptable.

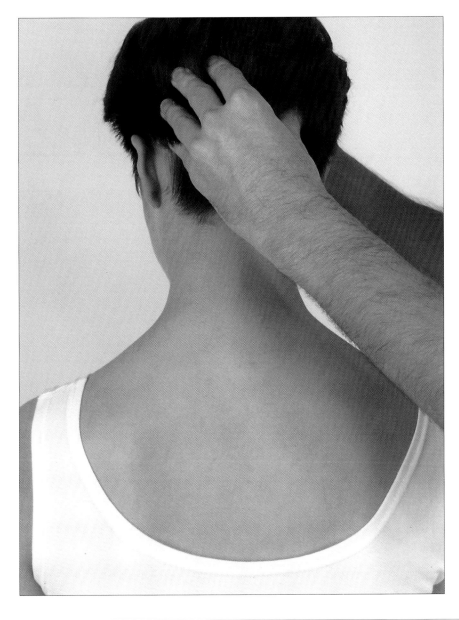

7c Continue the previous movement up onto the scalp. Press your fingers into the scalp and rotate them slowly. Use the pads of your middle three fingers. Remember to move the scalp under your fingers and not your fingers on the scalp. If the scalp is particularly tense it will not move easily. If this is the case, press deeply and rotate only where you can. The pressure will begin to relax the scalp and release the tightness. Work over as much of the head as you can reach. Then come to the other side of the body to repeat the previous two strokes and then this one. Proceed to stroke 8.

Common Ailments

Before you start to massage your partner, always ask if there are any physical problems. Here is a list of the most common neck and shoulder complaints you are likely to encounter and the best course of action in each case.

● **Frozen Shoulder**
This common condition is akin to Tennis Elbow and Golfer's Elbow. All three are likely to be inflamed and quite painful. You can help by using light effleurage. This encourages the circulation and movement of lymph. Working on the muscles around the joint will also reduce accumulated muscle tension.

● **Neck Stiffness and Shoulder Tension**
Both these common complaints will respond to the neck-and-shoulder sequence, particularly kneading the shoulders using the two-handed stroke (see page 37). A stiff neck will respond well to kneading on the neck and the finger work up the sides of the neck.

● **Repetitive Strain Injury (RSI)**
This condition is caused by repetitive physical stress on various areas of the body and exacerbated by bad posture. In this situation it is best to advise your partner to see a physiotherapist. I have found however, that the neck-and-shoulders sequence is beneficial in helping reduce muscle fatigue and ache in cases of RSI.

● **Tension Headaches**
Often caused by neck stiffness, they can be helped by releasing the neck.

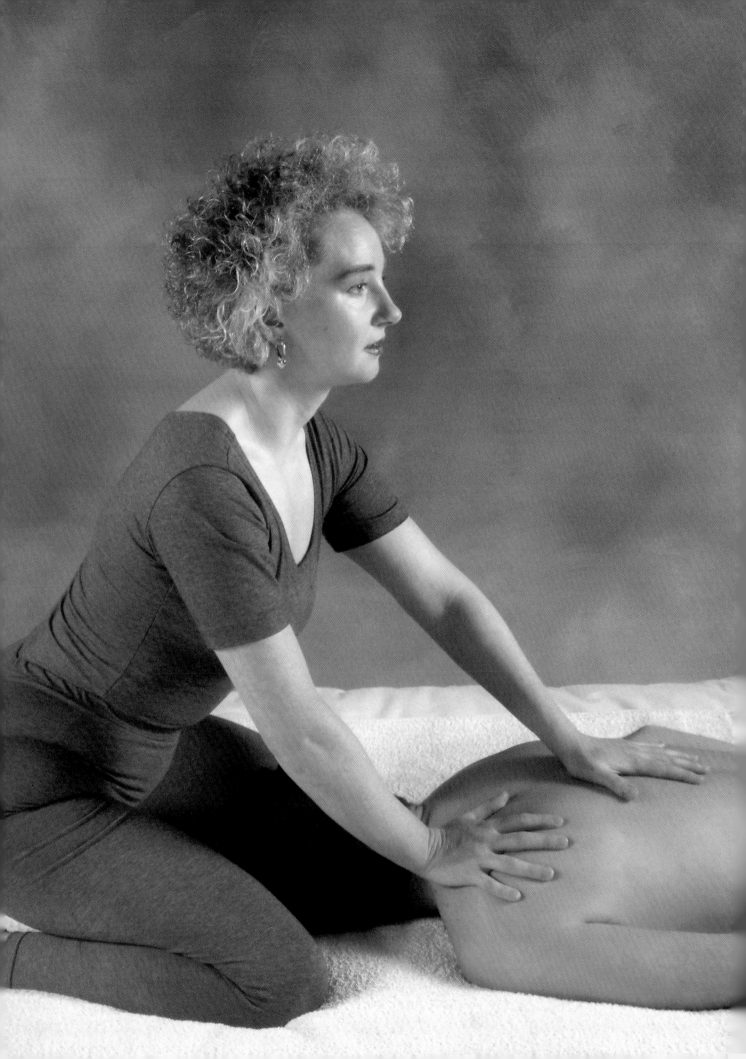

2

Back and Buttocks

The back is a wonderful area on which to give and receive massage. It is a very 'safe' part of the body, as it is much more protected than, for example, the chest or abdomen. A good back massage will not only leave the back feeling relaxed and energized, but the whole body will enjoy the effect. If only one area of the body is to be massaged, then the back is certainly the most effective.

The back is extremely vulnerable. Back pain accounts for more lost working days than any other complaint. Mental and emotional turmoil also lodges here. The back is a means of support, and we associate it with character and integrity.

The buttocks store inordinate amounts of tension. It is here that we house our unexpressed anger and fear, unconsciously clenching the buttocks together to hold on to such emotions. We are all familiar with the proverbial 'anal retentive' personality who is rigid, uptight and has difficulty relaxing. Such a person is also likely to be guarded, unyielding and ungenerous in sharing emotions, possessions and definitely his or her money. This is clearly because this type of person feels unsupported and essentially unloved. They trust no-one and keep other people at a distance. Caring touch will disperse this type of apprehension, infusing a person with sympathy and reassurance.

Conversely, it is probably unwise to massage this type of person's buttocks until he or she feels very comfortable with you. It is quite enough to work on the rest of the body until this time. When you do massage the buttocks, however, the recipient will feel a huge difference within, experiencing a sense of lightness, both physically and emotionally.

The back is the largest surface area you will work on. It is the ideal place to learn many of the strokes you will use elsewhere on the body.

41

Back and Buttocks

The back and buttocks area includes the spinal column and the pelvis as well as the overlying muscles. The spinal column consists of thirty-three bones known as vertebrae, some of which fuse together to form the sacrum and coccyx. The vertebrae are linked together by the intervertebral discs and small synovial joints to allow the spinal column to be both a supportive and mobile structure.

The top of the spine comprises the cervical region – the neck vertebrae – and the thoracic area – the upper-back region – to which the rib-cage is attached. It continues into the lumbar or lower-back area and the sacrum, which forms the central portion of the pelvis, the remainder of which is formed by the hip bones.

Viewed from the side, the spine is structured as in a series of curves that flow from one region to the next. These curves provide the spine with flexibility, allowing it to act as a shock absorber. Abnormalities in these curves may lead to problems such as kyphosis, scoliosis and lordosis. Kyphosis is an exaggerated curve in the thoracic spine resulting in the classic 'dowager's hump' appearance. Scoliosis is a sideways curvature of the spine, while lordosis is an increased inwards curve in the lower back. These conditions all limit the movement of the spine and decrease its capacity to absorb shock.

The spinal cord lies within the spine and houses the central nervous system. Here the nerves are formed that supply the peripheral parts of the body. The spinal cord provides a direct connection between the brain and the rest of the body. Nerves conveying impulses from the brain to the various organs and tissues descend through the spinal cord. Similarly, sensory nerves from organs and tissues enter and pass upwards to the brain via the spinal cord. Massage on the back gives access to the workings of the entire body through its direct action on the spinal nerves. It relaxes and tones these nerves, improving the condition of all the organs.

THE BACK AND BUTTOCKS MUSCLES EXPLAINED

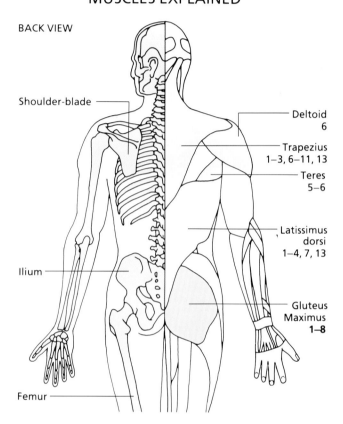

BACK VIEW

Shoulder-blade

Ilium

Femur

Deltoid
6

Trapezius
1–3, 6–11, 13

Teres
5–6

Latissimus
dorsi
1–4, 7, 13

Gluteus
Maximus
1–8

Numbers refer to steps in the following sequence, showing at which stage each muscle is worked upon. Numbers in bold type apply to the second sequence in this lesson.

The back is covered with large muscles, many of which connect the spine to the limbs. The main ones that are worked on in this chapter are illustrated here. One of the largest of the back muscles is the trapezius, a flat muscle that extends from the base of the skull to the lower thoracic region of the spine and inserts into the shoulder-blade. The trapezius is often a site of tension, causing discomfort in the neck, shoulder and upper back. The deltoid muscle connects the collar-bone and shoulder-blade to the humerus and makes the shoulder rounded. The teres muscles also connect these bones. Lower on the back lies the latissimus dorsi. The Gluteus Maximus rises from the back of the pelvis, the ilium of which can be seen here, and crosses the hip to insert into the femur.

Back

The following back sequence is your first opportunity to work directly on the skin. A large, flat surface area, the back is ideal for practising on to gain confidence. Many of the strokes you encounter in this sequence will be applied to smaller areas of the body later on, so gaining experience with them on this larger area is of great benefit.

People who are unaccustomed to receiving massage generally prefer their back to be worked on as it is the area they feel least inhibited about revealing. As a beginner myself, many years ago, I spent my early apprenticeship working on backs. I never encountered anyone who was at all reserved about volunteering his or her back for me to practise on. Had I been requesting the front of the body, I might not have been met with such unanimous enthusiasm.

Another good reason for beginning on the back is that your partner is not directly facing you. He is more able to relax and less likely to feel awkward and obliged to chat. Even when you are carrying out a complete body treatment, I would still recommend that you start on the back. When you are more familiar with giving massage and, more importantly, when your partner is more at ease with receiving massage from you, you may well choose to begin your treatment on the front of the body.

Before you start to massage the back, always make sure that your partner is in the correct position. The back is a large surface area so you will need to be able to reach all of it comfortably. To do this, place your partner's arms out to the sides of his body. This simple movement will give you room to kneel comfortably alongside him. Make sure that you do not lean into him: this will be very uncomfortable and distracting for your partner. But do not kneel too far away either, as you will not be able to work effectively.

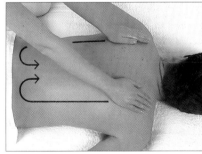

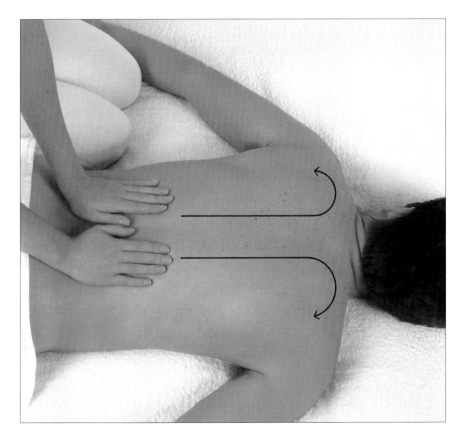

1 Apply the oil to your hands, away from your partner's body. Breathe in, and as you breathe out make contact. Begin to effleurage by gliding both hands up the back and around the shoulders (*see left*). Draw hands lightly down the sides of the back to the starting position (*see above*). The dynamic here is on the upward motion towards the heart with light contact on the return stroke. Lean your body into your hands to apply more pressure. You can come up on your knees but keep the pressure steady. Repeat this four to five times.

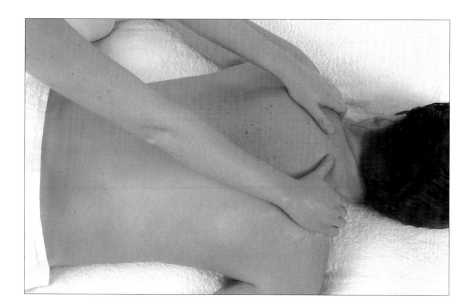

2 Glide hands up the back exactly as you have just done in step 1. Extend hands over the shoulders, hook fingers into the front of the shoulder muscles and pull back, leaning your body for maximum effect (*see top right*). The return stroke uses only the sides of the hands for very light contact, opening the hands out as shown here (*see middle right*). Repeat twice.

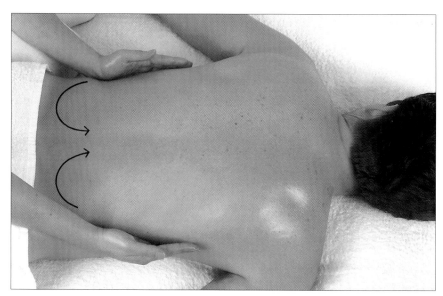

3 Place hands on the lower back as if you were beginning to effleurage. Push hands out to the sides of the body, circling them around and back to meet each other. Continue the stroke, moving up the back with each set of circles until you reach the shoulders. Draw the hands down to the lower back using the sides of your hands as in step 2.

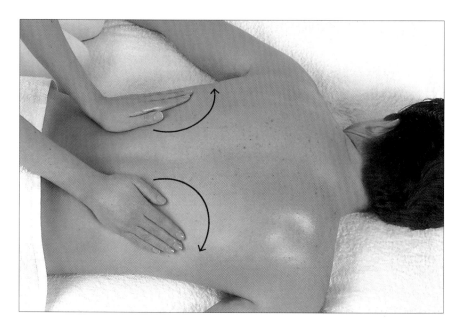

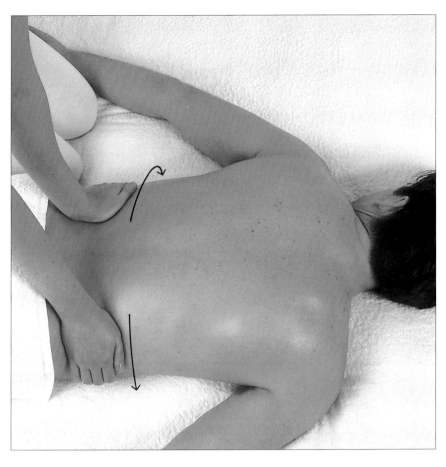

4 Place hands on lower back, fingers facing away from each other. Begin to petrissage by leaning heels of hands into the groove either side of the spine and pushing heels towards your fingers. Do not allow the fingers to glide down the back. Work up the back to the shoulder-blades, decreasing the pressure as you work over the kidney area.

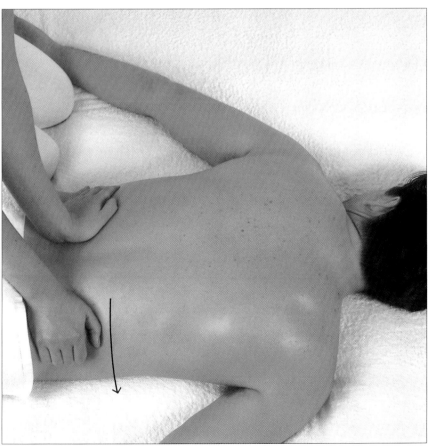

5 The petrissage stroke described in step 4 should now be applied to one side of the spine at a time. Keep both hands parallel, resting one alongside the other as it works. This makes the stroke much more focused and efficient. You need to work on the side furthest away from you, so when you have completed one side, move to the other side of your partner's body and carry out the stroke from there. Work up to the shoulder blades. When finished, stay on this side to carry out strokes 6, 7, 8, 9 and 10 and then move back to repeat them on the other side.

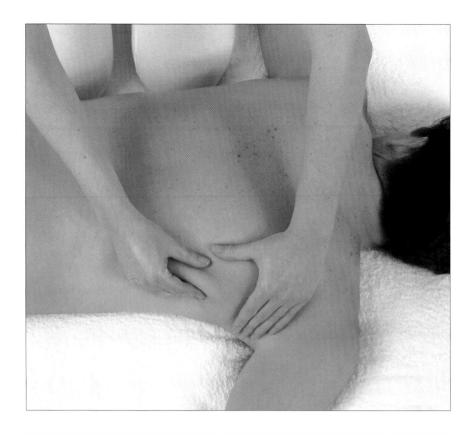

6 Check the position of your partner's arm, moving it gently if you need more room. Move your body so that your knees are facing your partner's back. Begin to knead by pushing one hand into the muscle just below the armpit, picking up flesh and squeezing it between fingers and thumb. Then move the other hand in exactly the same way. Set up an even rhythm with one hand starting as the other is finishing. Repeat four to five times.

7 Move your knees to face the opposite shoulder-blade. Begin to effluerage by placing both hands on top of the shoulder-blade and pushing down towards the arm. Glide your hands in the direction of the arrows (*see right*). Use your body-weight to bring momentum into the movement. When you push over the shoulder-blade, come up onto your knees if necessary, but only if you can still control the pressure. Lean backwards using your full body-weight when you pull the hands back. Finish by resting your hands in opposite directions at the top of the shoulder-blade (*see below*). Stay on this side of the body for the next stroke.

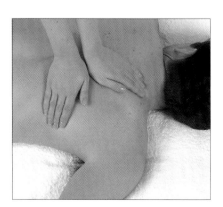

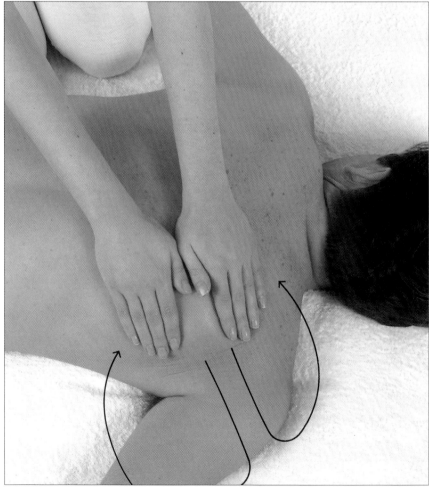

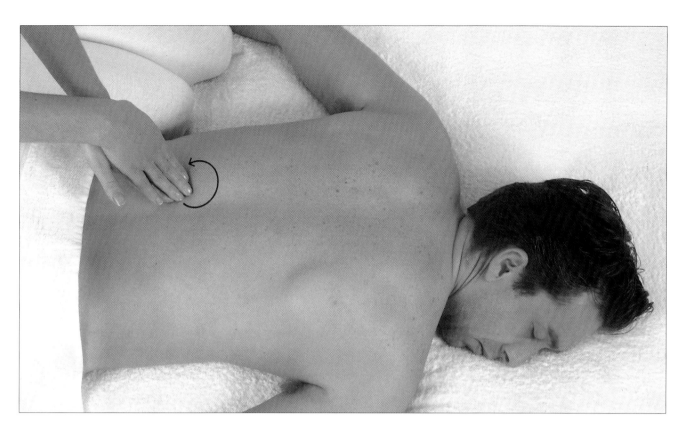

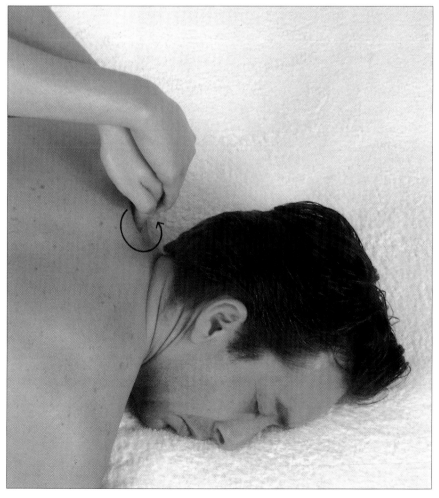

8 Return to your original position, kneeling alongside your partner. Work on the nearest side of the body. Place one hand on top of the other, fingers straight and pointed, in the groove next to the spine (*see above*). Lean the fingers into the groove and slowly rotate them on the muscle below. Do not bend your fingers. Continue working up the back in this way, applying and releasing pressure very gradually, until you reach the shoulder. For the next part of the stroke (*see left*) you may need to move your body closer to the shoulder. Apply the fingers in exactly the same way along the top of the shoulders, pressing into the muscle and rotating. Work from the inner shoulder near the neck to the outer. Repeat this stroke once. Stay on this side of the body for the next stroke.

47

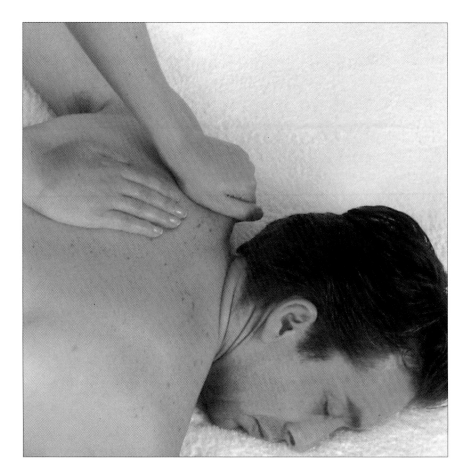

9 Move your body so you can comfortably reach the shoulder. Come up onto your knees and push the heel of one hand into the shoulder muscle, anchoring your hand by wrapping your fingers around the front of the shoulder. Continue to push the heel of hand into the muscle until the hand slips off the shoulder. Make sure you are using your full body-weight to push into and squeeze the muscle. Repeat four to five times using both hands alternately.

10 Maintain the same body position, up on your knees, leaning into the shoulders. Pick up the shoulder muscle between fingers and thumb, lean in and squeeze firmly. Support yourself with the other hand. Continue squeezing and push the thumb and heel of hand right off the shoulder. Repeat with the other hand. Unless you are working on a very large person and have lots of space, you will be able to work with only one hand at a time. Repeat four to five times. Now move to the other side of the body and take up your original position. Repeat the single-handed petrissage (step 5), kneading on the side of the body (step 6), effleurage on the shoulder-blade (step 7), friction work alongside the spine (step 8) and kneading the shoulder muscle (steps 9 and 10).

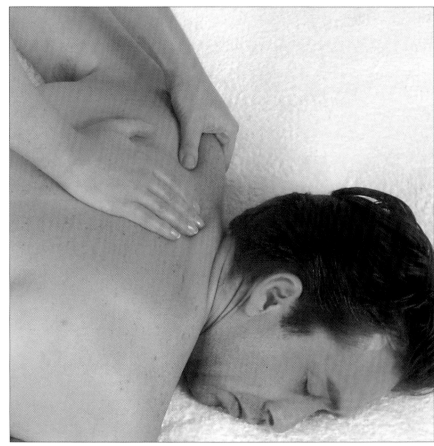

11 Ask your partner to rest his head on his hands. Position yourself comfortably with your body weight over the neck and head. Try placing your outside leg in front of you, foot parallel to your partner's head, inside leg kneeling up. Stabilize the head with one hand, while the other squeezes into the neck, working up towards the base of the skull (*see below*). Be careful not to let your thumb and forefinger slip around to the throat. Work up and down the neck two to three times.

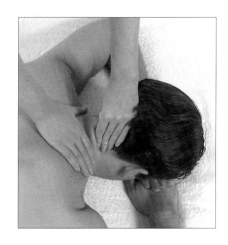

12 As a variation on step 11, squeeze down the neck with one hand as the other squeezes up to meet it (*see above*). This kneading-squeezing action usually works better here with your thumb and fingertips rather than the whole hand. Do not irritate your partner by merely pinching the flesh. Work up and down the neck three to four times. When you are confident with the entire back routine, insert the Additional Sequence on pages 51–56 here.

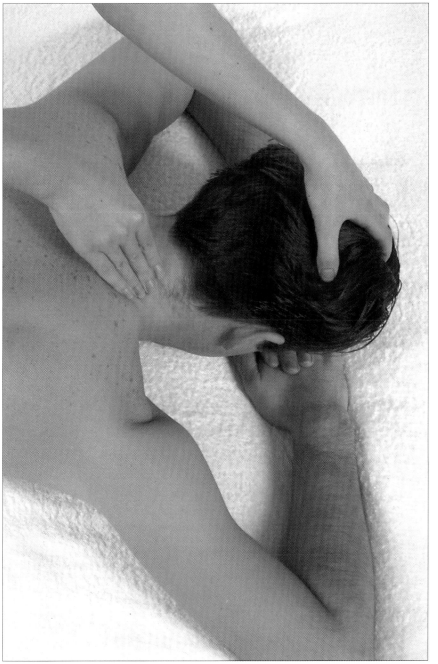

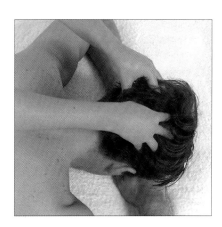

13 Place your fingertips on the head. Bend your fingers so that you increase the pressure. Press fingertips into the scalp and rotate slowly (*see above*). Press and rotate the fingers methodically all over the head. Pay special attention to the base of the skull. The area around the ears is also valuable, working here will release great amounts of tension. Aim to move the scalp underneath your fingertips. When finished, ask your partner to bring his hands down to his sides again.

14 Position yourself alongside your partner. Effleurage again by leaning your hands into the lower back, gliding up to and around the shoulders, down the sides of the body to the lower back. Repeat four to five times. You can finish with this stroke or continue with the next one. If you do finish here, 'ground' your partner.

15 Place your fingertips on the top of the back and draw them slowly down it one hand after the other. As one hand reaches the lower back, bring it to the top again immediately. Carry out the movement in this direction only. Lighten the contact gradually, so your touch is almost imperceptible. Some people will not respond well to this stroke, finding it irritating. If so, complete the back sequence with step 14. Put your partner's arms gently by his sides. Cover him up. 'Ground' him by holding his feet for at least 20 seconds.

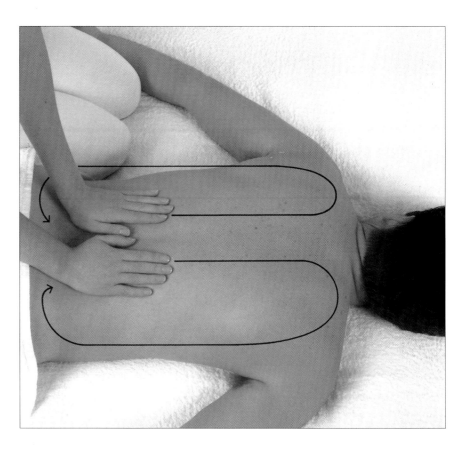

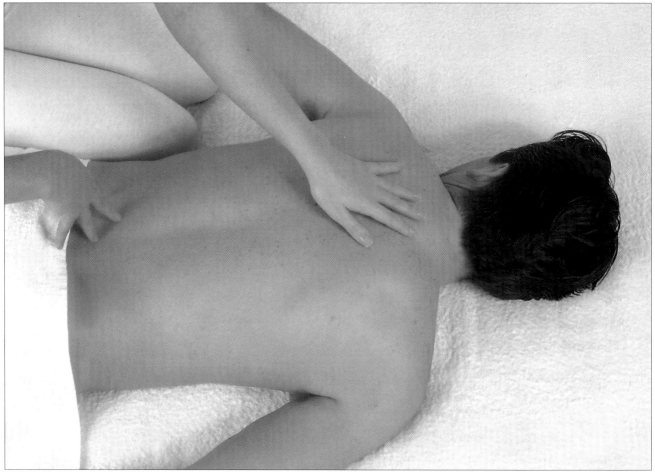

Additional Sequence

The following sequence for the back is thorough and complete in itself. Before attempting it, I recommend that you have practised the previous back sequence on at least three occasions for a minimum period of 20 minutes. When carrying out a full-body massage, or simply a back treatment, you can use this back sequence as an alternative to the one previously demonstrated. It differs from the previous sequence in that it concentrates particularly on the upper back and shoulder area. Many people suffer from discomfort, even pain, in this region, usually as a result of stress brought on by bad posture. If your partner needs concentrated massage here, you may choose to do this sequence.

You may like, alternatively, to do a thorough, extended back treatment by incorporating this additional work into the previous sequence. If this is the case, follow these guidelines. Stop the previous sequence after you have kneaded the neck (step 3). Bring your partner's arms alongside him and position yourself at the top of the body astride the head. It is most important that you position yourself neither too far away from nor too close to your partner's head. As a guide, position your knees parallel to his ears. You are now ready to start the additional sequence, which takes at least 15 minutes to complete thoroughly. Another reason why this is a particularly useful routine is that your position at the top of the body allows you to drop your full weight into your partner's body by leaning over it directly, thus giving potential for a deeper massage treatment to be carried out.

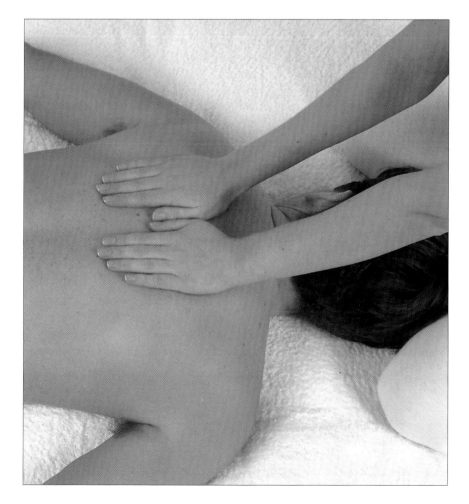

1 Position yourself astride your partner's head. Apply oil to your hands away from the body and make contact. Bring your awareness to the muscles beneath your hands. The upper back is a painful place for many people where muscles are usually held tightly and rigidly. If your touch here is warm, soothing and sympathetic you will help just by maintaining contact. Close your eyes and focus on any changes taking place in the body. It is quite likely that you will feel muscles twitching as they release their contracted position and relax. Stay here for at least 30 seconds.

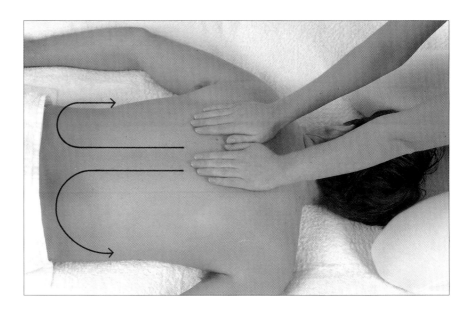

2 Place your hands on the upper back, either side of the spine (*see top right*). Breathe in. As you breathe out, lean your weight into your hands and push down until you reach the lower back. Make sure that all of your hand is in contact with the body. You can either lean forward with your arms while still kneeling, or for a much more dynamic effect, come up onto your knees and drop your weight into the stroke but check your shoulders are not hunching up. At the lower back, move your hands outwards and pull them up the sides of the body. At the armpit, pull your hands in towards the spine (*see middle right*). Draw your hands over the shoulder-blades (*see bottom right*). To repeat this stroke, simply bring your hands back to the starting position alongside each other. You may repeat this step four to five times. Alternatively, you can continue straight into step 3 by leaving your hands resting on your partner's shoulder-blades.

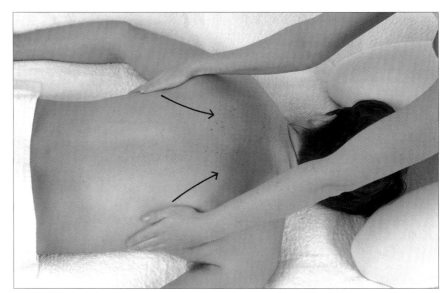

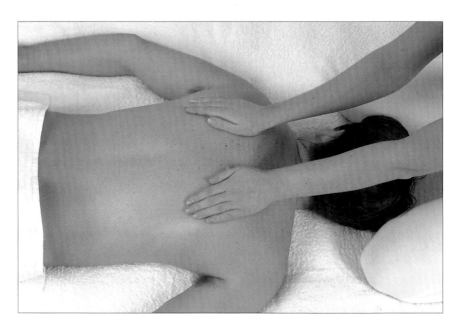

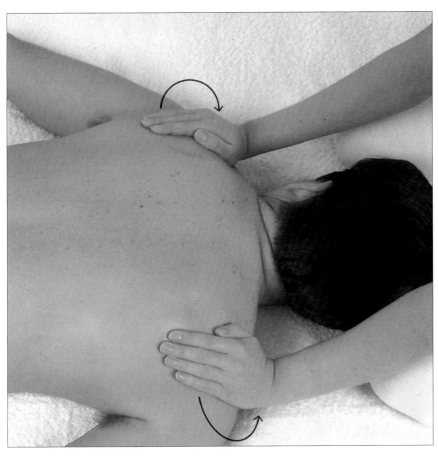

3 Continue to glide your hands up onto your partner's shoulder-blades and out towards his arms (*see left*). Scoop your hands around the shoulders. Continue this movement up onto the neck (*see below*) with the other hand resting on the shoulder nearest the face. Be very careful not to let your hand slip onto the throat or your partner's face. This can feel invasive or threatening at worst, and will at best disturb your partner. Repeat steps 2 and 3 twice.

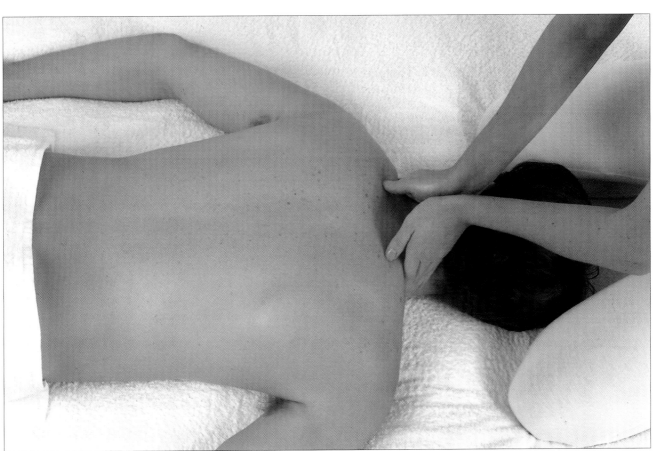

4 Place thumbs either side of the spine at the top of the back with fingers resting to the sides. Breathe in. As you breathe out, lean your weight into your thumbs and push down the back. Keep the fingers in contact with the back as a secure anchor for your thumbs. When your thumbs reach the shoulder-blades you will need to come up onto your knees to distribute your weight sufficiently for the rest of the stroke. At the lower back, glide hands up the sides of the back to move straight into the next stroke.

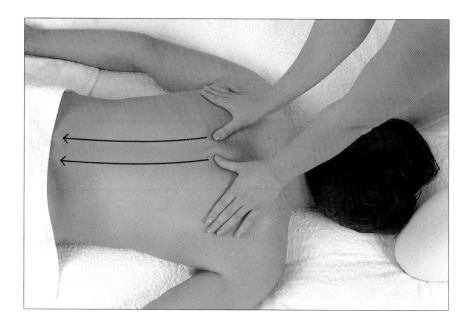

5 Rest one hand on the upper back and draw the other one around the edge of the shoulder-blade in the direction of the arrow (*see right*). Pull the hand back firmly towards the head. When you reach the shoulder, push the heel of your hand into and along the shoulder muscle out to the arm. Relax your fingers and concentrate solely on the heel of your hand. Rest this hand on the upper back as you repeat the stroke on the other side with the other hand. You can also do this stroke using both hands at once (*see below*). Place both hands on the upper back. Draw them back towards the head and push into and along the top of both shoulders with the heel of the hand.

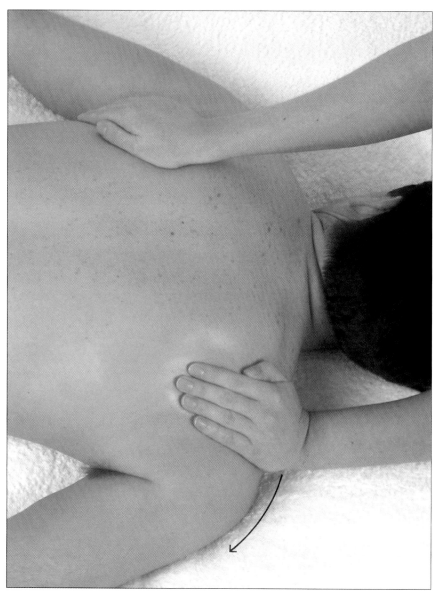

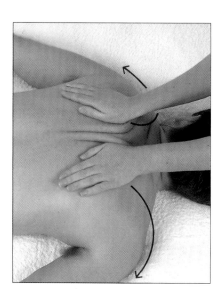

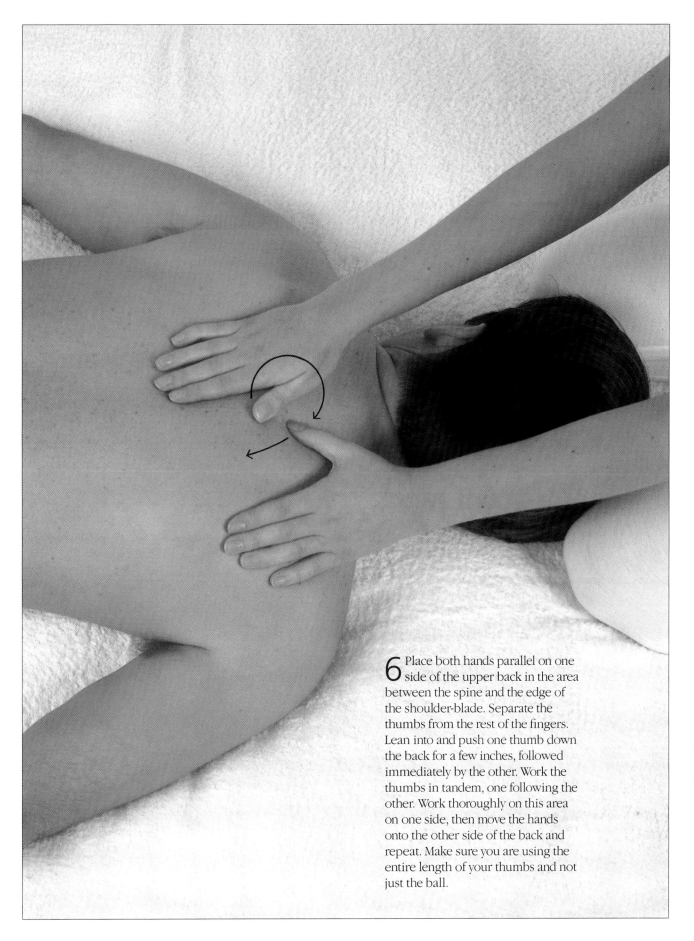

6 Place both hands parallel on one side of the upper back in the area between the spine and the edge of the shoulder-blade. Separate the thumbs from the rest of the fingers. Lean into and push one thumb down the back for a few inches, followed immediately by the other. Work the thumbs in tandem, one following the other. Work thoroughly on this area on one side, then move the hands onto the other side of the back and repeat. Make sure you are using the entire length of your thumbs and not just the ball.

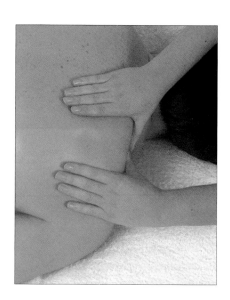

7 Bring both hands to work on one shoulder at a time. Place your thumbs lengthways along the top of the shoulder muscle (*see right*). Breathe in, and as you breathe out, lean your weight into your thumbs gliding along the muscle to the shoulder-joint. Repeat twice on this side. Bring your hands to the other side and repeat the movement, taking care to avoid your partner's face.

Finally, place your hands on both shoulders, beginning as close to the head as possible. Breathe in, and as you breathe out, lean your weight into your thumbs as they glide across the shoulders to the shoulder-joint (*see below*). Repeat twice. If you are using this sequence on its own, remember to 'ground' your partner by moving to the feet and holding them for at least 20 seconds.

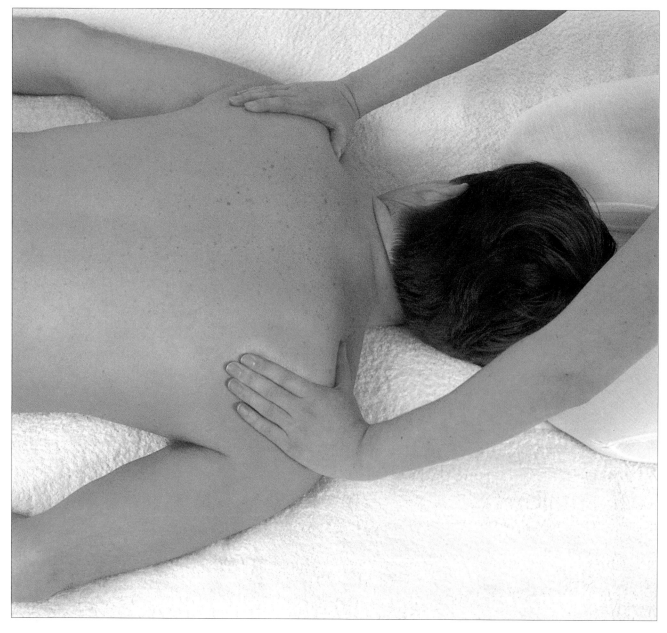

Buttocks

The buttocks are one of the most private and least-exposed areas of the body. It is the area least likely ever to receive touch, (even during a massage treatment). This is understandable. You should only include the following sequence when your partner is comfortable with receiving massage from you and is happy to have this area worked on.

The buttocks are nonetheless one of the most pleasant areas on which to receive a massage. The gluteus maximus muscles make up the bulk of the buttocks and can store enormous amounts of tension. It is important, then, to be especially confident in your touch when you massage here. When carrying out the petrissage strokes, work deeply and firmly. Once you are experienced, a treatment that does not include the buttocks will feel quite incomplete.

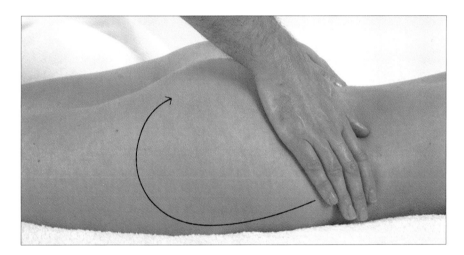

1 Make contact on the lower back. Begin to effleurage the buttock by gliding your hands away from each other, fingers pointing down towards the sides of the body (*see left*). Draw the hands around the sides of the buttocks in the direction of the arrow. Push up over the buttocks (*see below*) and return to the starting position. The pressure in this stroke is applied as you draw your hands around the sides of the buttocks and particularly as you push up and over towards the lower back. Repeat this movement four to five times.

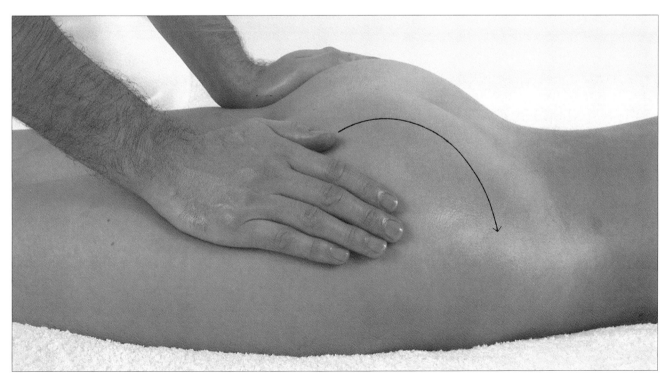

2 Move to face the buttock furthest from you. Push one hand into the buttock, scoop up the muscle between fingers and thumb and squeeze firmly. Repeat with the other hand. Introduce a flowing rhythm by moving your hands alternately. Knead well all over the buttock.

3 Beginning at the top, lean the heel of the hand into the buttock. As you push down, squeeze the muscle between heel of hand and fingers. Return to top and repeat with other hand. Continue to petrissage four or five times with alternate hands. Move to the other side of the body and repeat steps 2 and 3 on other buttock.

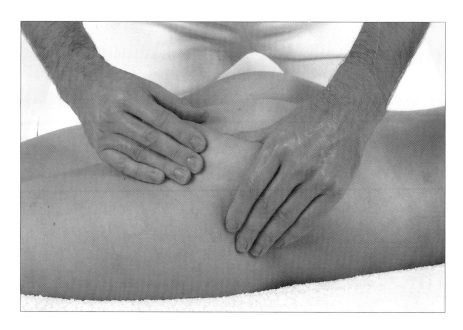

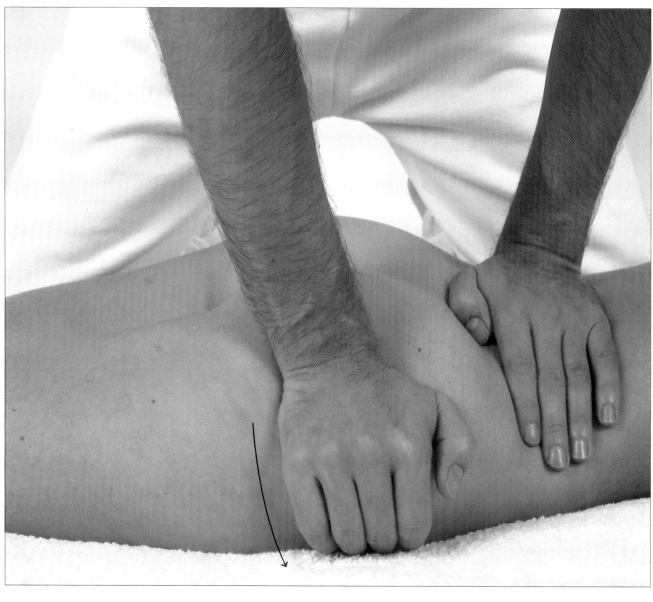

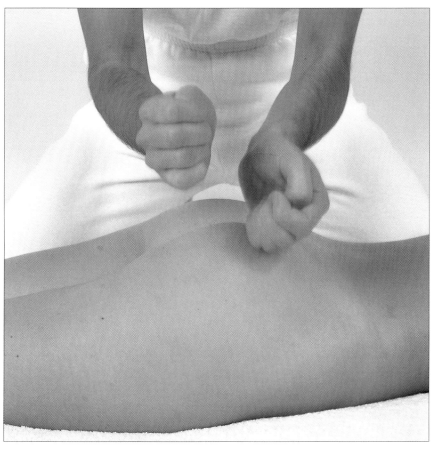

4 Make the transition to the percussive strokes smoothly by beginning the pummelling gently. Bounce the hands alternately on the buttock, moving over the entire area. Keep your hands low and close to the buttock at all times. Maintain an even pace, working faster only if you are able to keep up this rhythm. If you do speed up the stroke, check that your hands are still low. Remember to breathe thoroughly throughout this stroke and encourage your partner to do so as well.

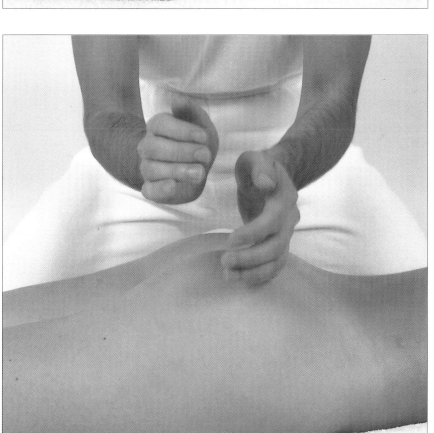

5 Make sure your wrists are relaxed before attempting this hacking stroke. Begin by hitting the buttock with the side of one hand followed immediately by the other hand. An even rhythm is imperative in hacking, more than any other stroke. Do the stroke slowly, increasing the speed only when you are thoroughly practised and adept at it. Work over the entire area equally and thoroughly. Encourage your partner to breathe and think of releasing tightness as the stroke breaks up long-standing tension.

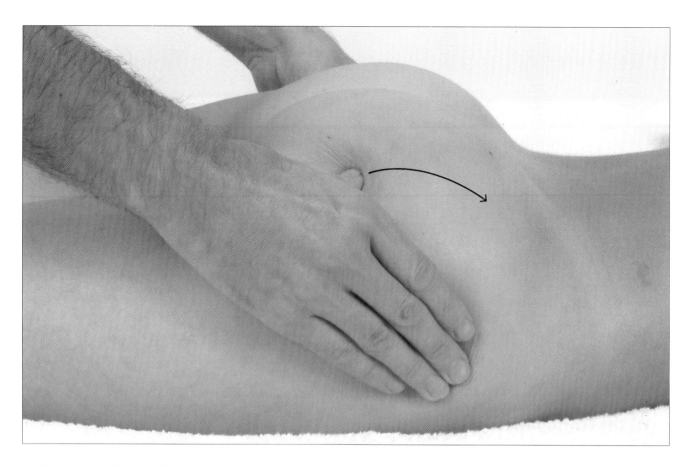

6 Imagine that there are three or four vertical lines running over each buttock from the top of the leg to lower back. Start with the 'line' on the side of buttock nearest you. Position your thumb on the leg just below the buttock. Anchor the rest of your hand on the side of the body (*see above*). Push in and glide thumbs up over the buttock towards the lower back. For more pressure, lean up on your knees, being particularly careful to keep the pressure steady. Return to starting point for each 'line'. Cover all 'lines' twice.

7 Point your hands, placing one on top of the other (*see right*). Keep your fingers straight and relaxed. Place the hands on the buttocks. Press the fingers into the muscles and rotate slowly. Work directly on the muscle; do not merely move the skin. Your pressure here is dictated by your partner's tolerance, but aim to work deeply. Work all over the buttock. It is imperative to apply and release the pressure gradually, avoiding abrupt movements.

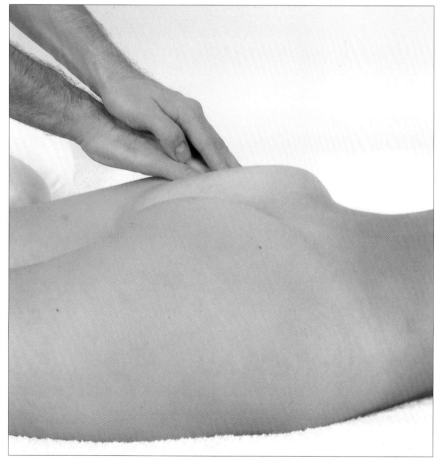

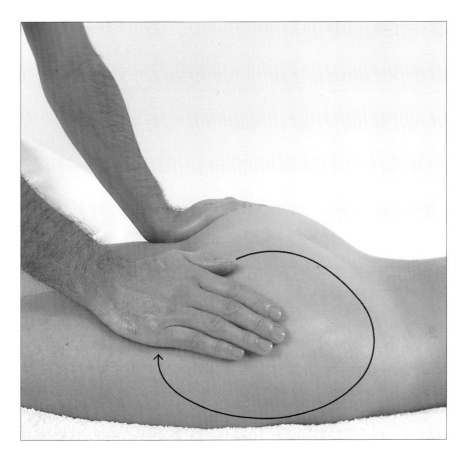

8 Begin a final effleurage stroke by placing your hands on the lower back, gliding out to the sides, back towards you and pushing up over the buttocks. Start this stroke lightly, gradually applying more pressure, particularly as you push up over the buttocks. As you finish, lessen the pressure until your touch is as light as when you began. Repeat the stroke at least four or five times. Effleurage at this point is particularly appreciated as it soothes the area after the deeper work and percussive strokes. 'Ground' your partner by holding the feet for at least 20 seconds.

Common Ailments

Before you start to massage your partner, always ask if there are any physical problems. Here is a list of the most common back complaints you are likely to encounter and the best course of action in each case: whether or not a massage would help and when medical attention is advisable.

● **Burning pain across shoulder-blades**
This is likely to be due to a build-up of toxins, accumulated as a result of poor circulation. Deep massage here with marjoram and lavender oils will be very useful.

● **Headaches**
These can arise from a combination of muscle tension and the constriction of blood flow to the head. Massage on the head (see page 49) and on the neck in particular will make a big difference. Oils of rosemary and

lavender will be helpful here.

● **Lower-backache**
This can manifest for a number of different reasons.

Ligament injury
The ligament can be torn by awkward lifting, whiplash or sudden twisting. The injury would be felt as a sharp pain or muscle spasm and generally restricted movement. Massage will help by increasing the circulation of blood and lymph to the area and relaxing the surrounding muscles. Lavender and marjoram are good oils here.

Post-pregnancy
Massage is of great benefit in relieving the compression and lower-back distortion brought on by pregnancy. It is important to have the back checked by a physiotherapist or osteopath after pregnancy and childbirth. Rose is a beautiful oil to use.

Pre-menstrual Tension
Prior to menstruation, it is quite common for women to be troubled with an aching lower back. Warming massage, particularly effleurage, is comforting and helpful. Use camomile or neroli oils.

● **Rheumatism**
Massage warms aching muscles and stimulates the circulation. Warming oils such as rosemary, juniper and ginger are useful.

● **Slipped Disc**
If one of the discs between the vertebrae becomes damaged through lifting or poor posture, then pressure may be caused by the jelly-like centre of the disc seeping out to impinge on the nerve and ligaments alongside the spine. Do not work on this serious condition, particularly if it is acute, with much pain and muscle spasm. Enlist a physiotherapist or osteopath.

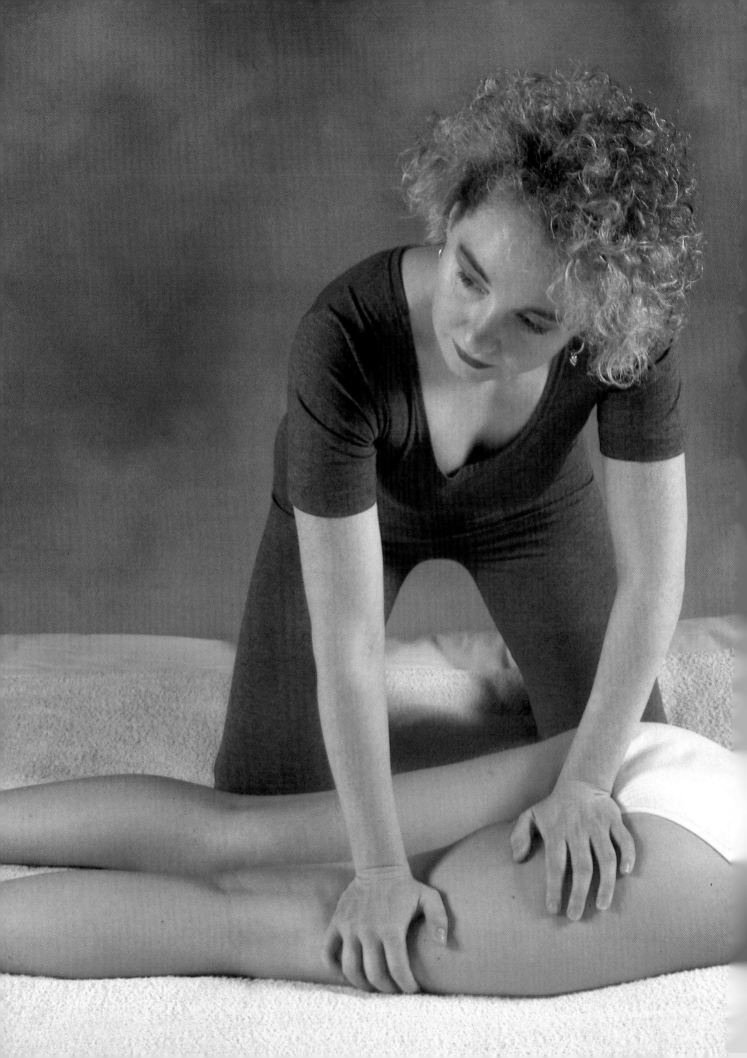

3

Back of Legs

T he backs of the legs are probably the most neglected area of the body. We rarely pay them any attention as they are difficult to see and reach. Yet our legs do us a great service, carrying the weight of our bodies around.

Standing or sitting still all day makes the circulation of blood and lymph literally an uphill struggle. Massage is of great benefit in assisting our circulation. Gentle effleurage up the legs helps to reduce water retention – around the ankles or in the thighs – and stimulates the flow of the lymph fluid at the back of the knees and in the groin.

Cellulite is a major health concern for many women. It suggests that the body cannot dispose of toxic waste materials. It also points to a sluggish lymphatic system that is not working efficiently enough to carry away the toxins that are trapped between the tissues in the fatty areas of the body, such as the buttocks and thighs. Combined with dietary changes and an exercise programme, massage is the only proven means of eradicating cellulite.

You need to use your body-weight very carefully in this sequence. Pressure on the calves, for example, must be applied sensitively and gradually, while pressure on the back of the knees is to be avoided at all costs. The thighs, on the other hand, need a great deal of pressure.

If you need to apply oil more than once when you initially effleurage the leg, stop, effleurage back down the leg, and re-oil your hands. This prevents you dragging the skin. Likewise, if your partner's leg is particularly hairy, use a lot more oil to avoid pulling the hair.

A good massage on the back of the legs can be a wonderful surprise. Relaxing and invigorating, it releases tension we may not have been aware of.

Back of Legs

When we are walking, the muscles in the back of the legs are responsible for moving the body along. Not surprisingly, these muscles are large and powerful. Many people have chronically tight calf and hamstring muscles. Massage will help to alleviate much of this tension, which people are often unaware of before they receive massage treatment.

At the hip there is a mobile ball-and-socket joint, where the femur – or thigh bone – meets the hip bone. Unlike the shoulder joint, it is protected by strong ligaments and has powerful muscles acting across it.

At the lower end of the femur is the knee joint. One group of three muscles, the hamstrings, lies between the hip and knee joints. Together they extend the hip and flex the knee, propelling the body in activities such as walking and running. They differ from the Gluteus Maximus muscle in the hip because they act more powerfully in activities where the knee is extended, in contrast to activities where the action of the gluteal muscles is more important, climbing the stairs, for example.

Tightness in the hamstrings restricts mobility at the hip, thereby increasing the strain on the lumbar spine, which may produce problems in the lower back. Back pain can sometimes be felt in the back of the legs. This is known as sciatica and may be confused with the pain of a hamstring injury.

The bones of the lower leg are the tibia and fibula. The tibia articulates with the femur to form the knee joint, and with the bones of the foot to form the ankle joint. There are deep and superficial muscles in this area. The gastrocnemius and the soleus are the most superficial. The bulk of the gastrocnemius muscle can be seen in the large, rounded calf muscle; the soleus lies beneath it. Both these muscles are inserted into the heel bone through the Achilles Tendon. The gastrocnemius muscle acts on the knee and the ankle joint, and is used powerfully in propulsive activities, especially jumping. A number of smal-

THE BACK OF LEGS MUSCLES EXPLAINED

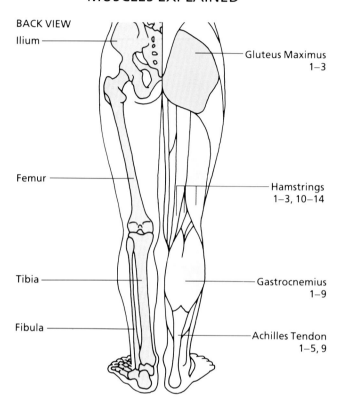

BACK VIEW
Ilium
Gluteus Maximus 1–3
Femur
Hamstrings 1–3, 10–14
Tibia
Gastrocnemius 1–9
Fibula
Achilles Tendon 1–5, 9

Numbers refer to steps in the following sequence, showing at which stage each muscle is worked upon.

The Gluteus Maximus and the hamstrings are powerful, propulsive muscles. They lie across the back of the pelvis, the ilium portion of which is shown above, and the femur. The Gluteus muscle forms the curve of the buttock and crosses the hip. The hamstrings cross the hip and knee. Below the knee, lying over the tibia and fibula, you can see the two bulky heads of the gastrocnemius or calf muscle. In the mid-calf region this muscle becomes the Achilles Tendon, which then passes down to insert, finally, into the heel.

ler muscles that act on the foot and toes lie even deeper. These muscles are used in walking.

Many of us spend our days engaged in sedentary activities, such as office work. Even leisure time can involve a great deal of sitting, such as watching television, eating out or spending an evening at the cinema. Such activities keep the muscles at the back of the leg, particularly the hamstrings, in a shortened state.

The body is an adaptable structure. If any muscle is not used throughout its full range, the soft tissue is likely to become even softer. This will create problems by restricting movement still further. It is not only people leading sedentary lives who suffer from this complaint but also athletes. Although they exercise their muscles vigorously, they must be careful to use them throughout their range of movement or problems will occur.

Massage can be of enormous benefit to people suffering in this way. It reduces tension in the muscles, which facilitates stretching. Deep massage on the entire back of the leg combined with stretching exercises will bring about profound change. The muscle fibres will lengthen, which can actually change the appearance of the leg, giving it a leaner look.

Athletes should always ensure that they warm up by carrying out some stretching exercises. If they do not, then there may be problems with knee extension due to an imbalance between the hamstring and quadriceps muscles.

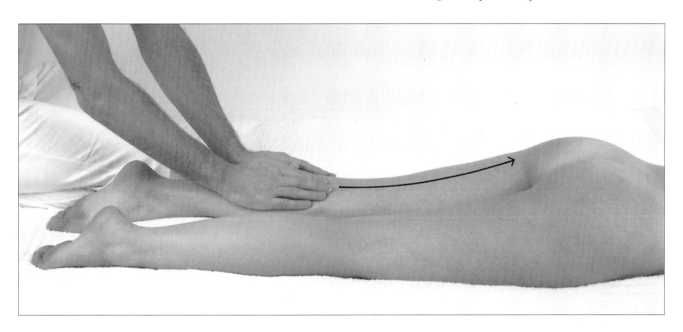

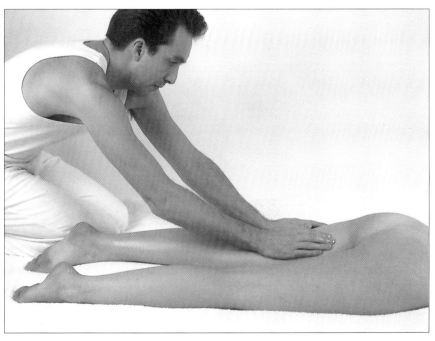

1 Apply the oil to your hands. Kneeling beside the feet, make contact, bringing your hands to rest gently on the leg, just above the ankle. Breathe in, and as you breathe out, smooth your hands up the leg (*see above*). Keep the pressure light and glide very lightly over the back of the knee. Reapply pressure as soon as you move beyond the knee into the thigh (*see left*). If you have difficulty reaching the upper thigh, lean up on your knees, keeping your feet firmly anchored on the floor. As your hands reach the top of the thigh, wrap your outside hand up and around the buttock in a smooth sweep, keeping the pressure firm. Be careful not to extend your inside hand too far up the inside thigh as this could feel invasive. Err on the side of caution.

2 From the top of the thigh, draw your hands down the sides of the leg keeping the pressure light. Remember to avoid any pressure on the back of the knee. As you reach the calf, squeeze the muscle between the heels of your hands (*see right*). Repeat this entire effleurage movement twice.

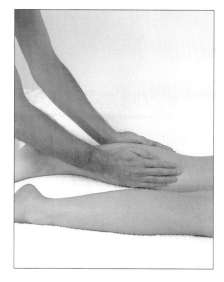

3 Place your hands on the lower leg, in a cupped position, with your fingers pointing in opposite directions (*see below*). Breathe in, and as you breathe out, lean gently into your hands as they glide slowly up the leg. As you reach the sensitive area at the back of the knee, take the pressure off and glide lightly onto the thigh, reapplying the pressure as soon as you have cleared the knee. Maintain your hands in this cupped position on the thigh, sweeping firmly around the buttock with your outside hand. Then complete this stroke by drawing both hands lightly down the leg to the ankle.

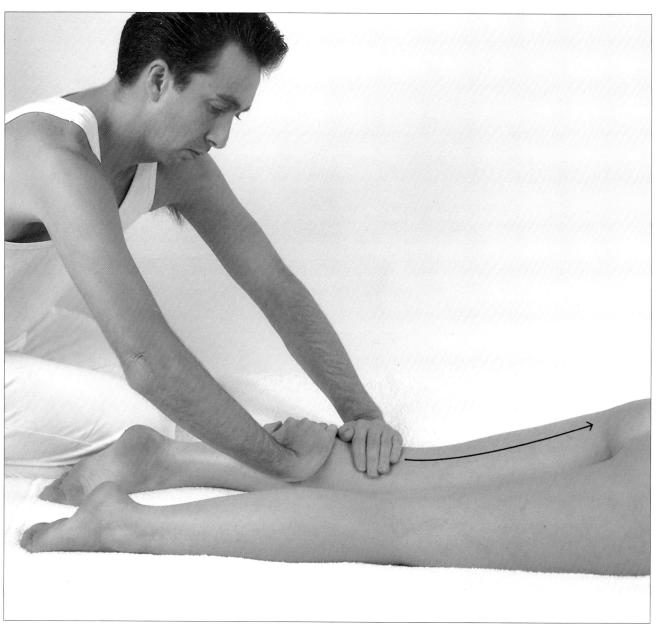

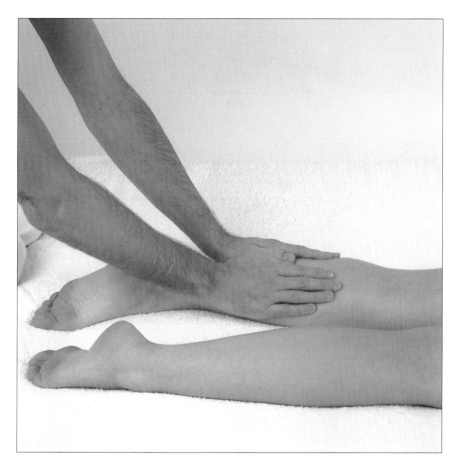

4 Place your hands flat on the lower leg. Breathe in, and as you breathe out, push your hands up the calf as far as the knee. Here, pull your hands back to the ankle again. As you have already warmed the muscles with the opening effleurage strokes, you can apply more pressure here. Take the pressure off as you reach the back of the knee.

5 Wrap your hands around the calf, just above the ankle. Breathe in, and as you breathe out, lean your weight into your hands to push up the calf as far as the knee. Lightly, draw your hands down the sides of the calf to the ankle.

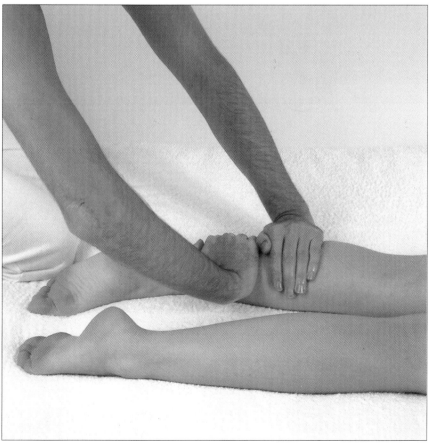

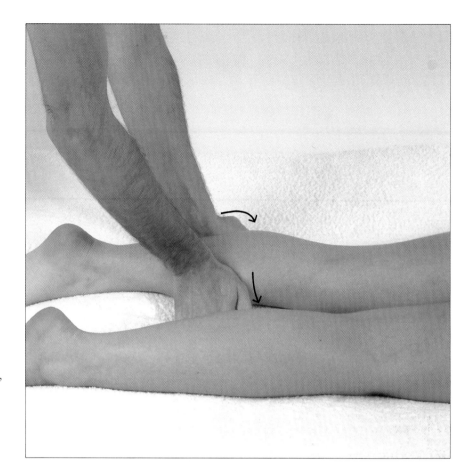

6 Place both hands on the calf just above the ankle, heels of hands next to each other, fingers wrapped around the front of the leg. Breathe in, and as you breathe out, lean into the heels of your hands, pushing them apart, away from each other and off the leg. Repeat this stroke up the calf until you reach the knee.

7 Rest one hand on the ankle. Position the other as for the previous stroke. Lean the heel of your hand into the calf and push sideways in the direction of your fingers, keeping them firmly in place. Continue the stroke until you have covered this half of the calf. Switch hands and continue the stroke with your other hand.

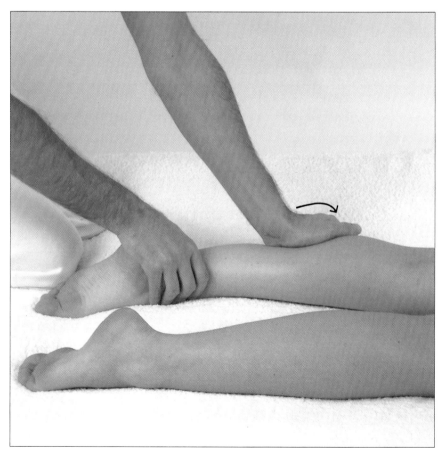

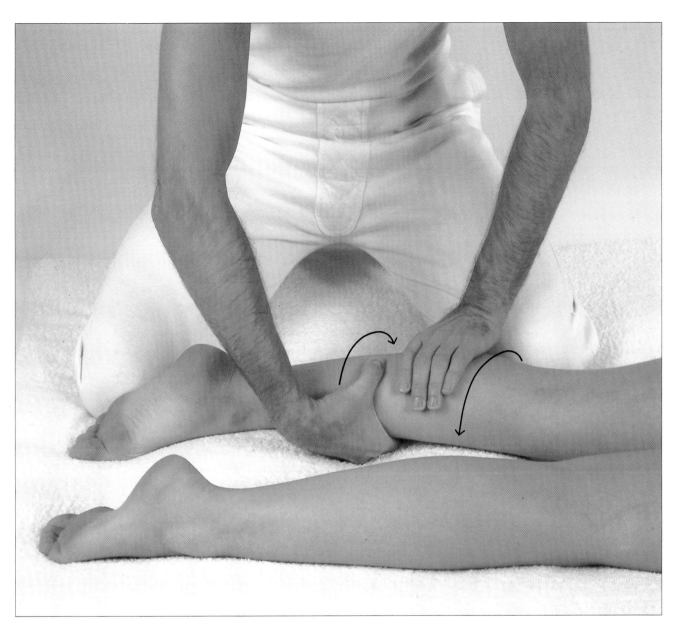

8 Change your position so you are facing your partner's calf. Wrap your hands around it in opposite directions, embracing the muscles between your thumb and fingers. Pull one hand towards you and at the same time push your other hand away from you. Keep a firm clasp on the muscles as you do this to ensure that your stroke is really dynamic and not merely another gliding movement. Aim to see the muscles lifted up and twisted as your hands move to and fro. Continue the movement until you have worked over the entire calf. You can now include a kneading stroke (*see page 74*) or continue straight on.

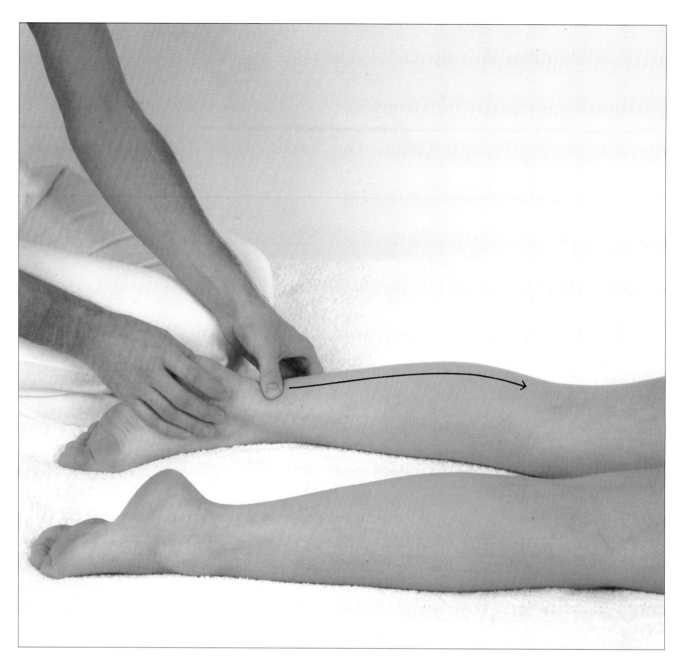

9 Return to your former position so that you are kneeling alongside the ankle. Rest one hand on the ankle. Wrap your other hand around the leg leaving your thumb free to rest on the centre of the calf. Place your thumb down flat (*see above*). Breathe in, and as you breathe out, lean slightly into your thumb as you glide it up the centre of the calf as far as the knee (*see right*). Apply very slight pressure to begin with, as this is a tense area for most people and you are focusing your thumb to work in a very concentrated way. Swap hands and repeat with your other thumb.

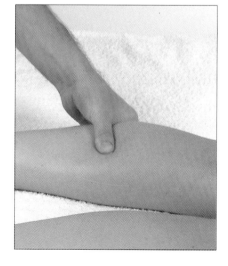

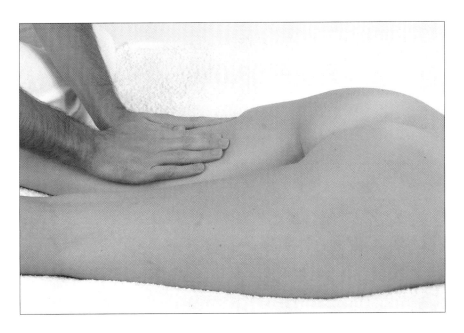

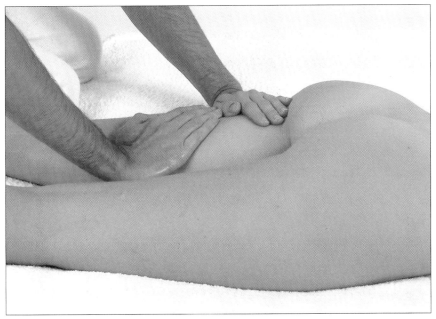

10 Move further up the body to kneel by your partner's knees. Place your hands gently on her thigh, just above the knee. Breathe in, and as you breathe out, lean your body weight into your hands as you push up the leg (*see top left*). For extra weight, come up on your knees, but do keep your feet on the ground to ensure your pressure is steady and secure. When you reach the top of the thigh, turn your hands (*see middle left*) and glide down to the knee. It is very important to respect your partner's privacy and not to work too far up the inside leg.

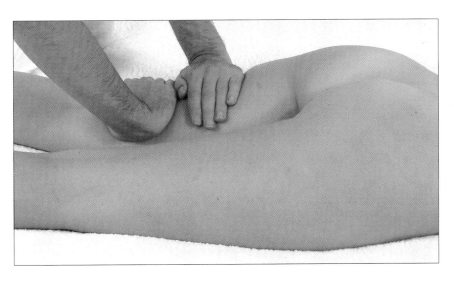

11 Position your hands, cupped around the thigh. Breathe in, and as you breathe out, lean into your hands as you push up the thigh. It usually feels very good if you can apply a lot of weight here. At the top of the thigh, push your outside hand up and over the buttock, maintaining the pressure, and pull it down the outside of the thigh, drawing your inside hand down the inside of the thigh at the same time.

71

12 Lean up on your knees and position your hands together with the heels touching and fingers wrapped around the front of the thigh as in step 6. Breathe in, and as you breathe out, lean into the heels of your hands as they push away from each other and off the thigh. Repeat until you have worked up the entire thigh.

13 Rest one hand on the thigh. Lean into the thigh with your other hand and push the heel sideways towards your fingers. Keep your fingers firmly in place so that you squeeze the flesh and muscles. Continue up the outside thigh, change hands and repeat on the inside thigh. You can now include a knuckling stroke (*see page* 75) or continue on to step 14.

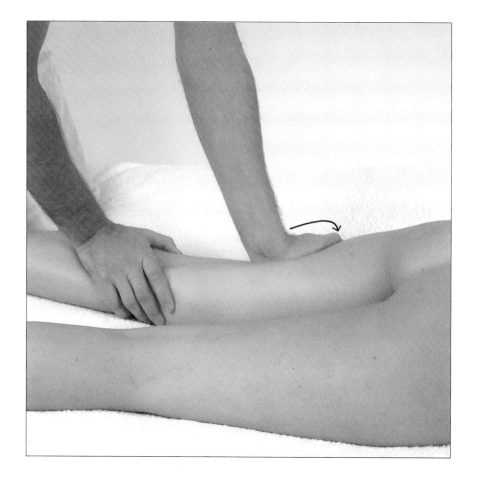

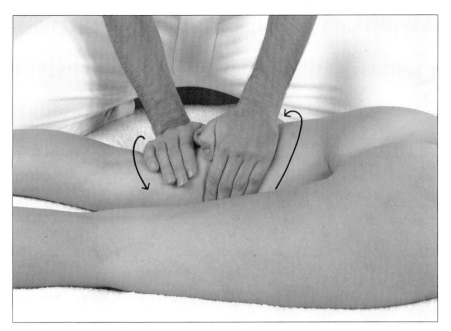

14 Face your partner's thigh. Place both hands parallel on the thigh. Push one hand away from you, pulling the other back towards you as you do this. This wringing movement needs to be very dynamic as the thigh is well padded. Aim to lift the muscle as you pull your hand back towards you, and use your body to lean into the push away. Do the stroke slowly until you are satisfied that you really are lifting, squeezing and wringing the muscle. Continue the movement until you have worked thoroughly up the thigh. You can now move on to a kneading stroke (*see page 74*) or the buttocks (*see pages 76 and 77*) or continue straight on to repeat the entire sequence on the other leg.

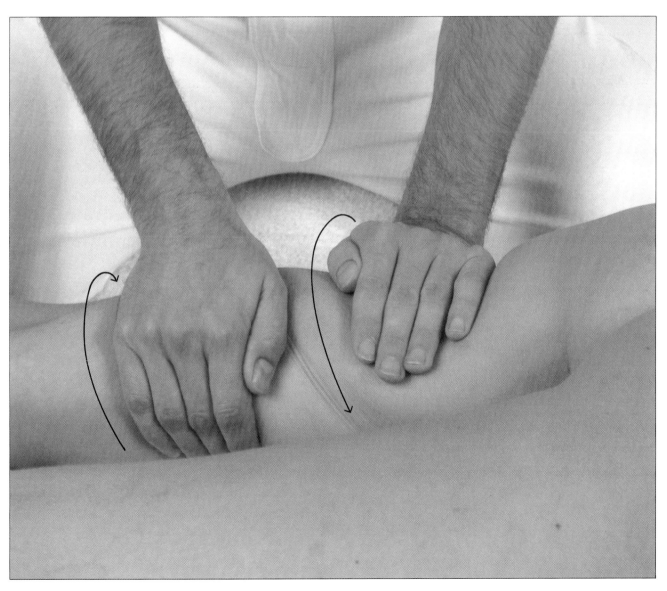

Additional Steps

The kneading strokes can enhance the back-of-legs routine immeasurably, squeezing out deep-seated tension and congestion. Women who suffer from cellulite or fluid retention will welcome the extra work on the thighs. Include kneading after step 8 (*see page 69*). Kneading on the thigh follows step 14 (*see page 73*).

The knuckling strokes are extremely powerful in stimulating movement and circulation in the area. Work them into your routine after you have completed all the kneading on the thigh or at least before the wringing movements in step 14 (*see page 73*).

Massaging the buttocks (*see pages 76–77*) is useful, as long as both you and your partner feel comfortable about it. You may move on to this area when you have finished all the other strokes. Work on the buttock furthest from you covering the buttock nearest you with a towel.

8a Move directly into this stroke when you have completed the wringing. Position your hands on the calf facing each other (*see right*). Lean in with one hand, lift and squeeze the muscle between fingers and thumb. Push towards the other hand as you repeat the movement with your other hand. Keep the movement flowing, slow and thorough as you cover the whole calf.

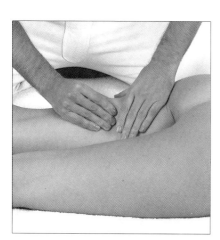

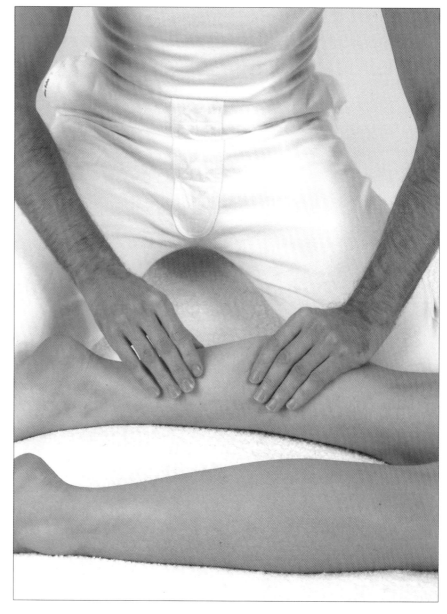

14a Place your hands on the thigh facing each other. Breathe in and as you breathe out, lean into one hand to lift up and squeeze the flesh between fingers and thumb (*see above*). Push towards your other hand. Lean in with the opposite hand to lift, squeeze and push. Begin the movement with your second hand as your first hand is completing so you set up a rhythm.

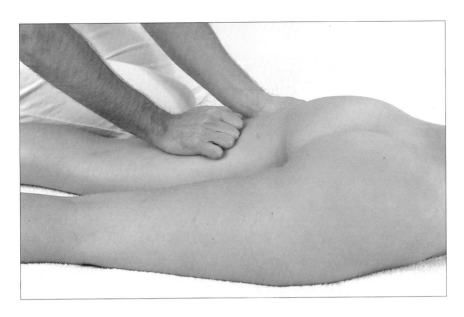

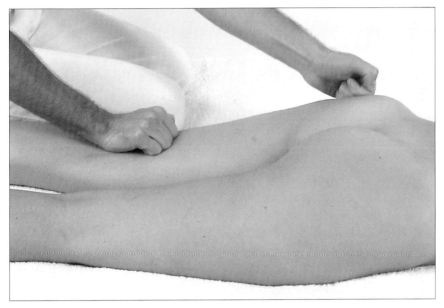

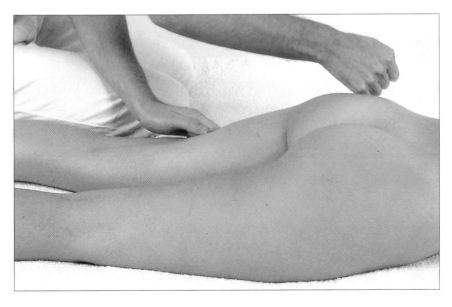

13a Make your hands into relaxed fists and rest them on the thigh (*see top left*). Lean slightly into your hands and run your knuckles up the inside of the thigh, one hand after the other. As always, do not work too far up the inside thigh. Repeat exactly the same movement on the centre of the thigh (*see middle left*). Work up to the buttock and bring your hands back to the starting position to repeat. Gradually bring your hands around to the outside of the thigh (*see bottom left*). Continue the movement up on to the buttock where you can really lean in deeply. The outside of the leg is usually quite a sensitive area, especially if there is congestion, so work quite lightly to begin with, gradually increasing the depth of pressure with your partner's co-operation. In this sequence you can choose either to give slow and thorough strokes or faster and more vigorous ones to achieve a more stimulating effect.

15 Work on the buttocks can help lower-backache and menstrual cramps. Lean up on your knees to enable you to drop your weight into the stroke. Place both hands flat on the buttock furthest from you. Breathe in, and as you breathe out, push into the buttock with the heel of your hand. Push towards your fingers and squeeze the flesh and muscle between the heel of your hand and your fingers. As soon as you have completed the stroke with one hand, begin with the other hand. Repeat the movements rhythmically at least five times with each hand. Include the other buttock after working on the other leg.

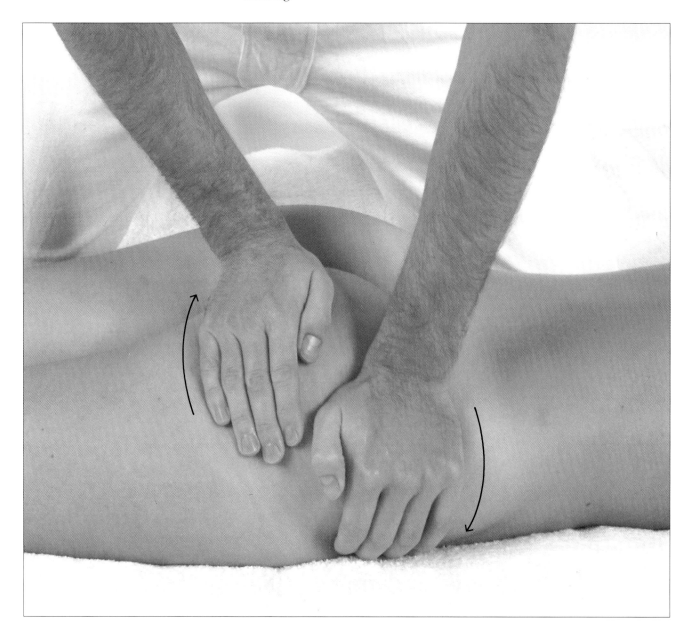

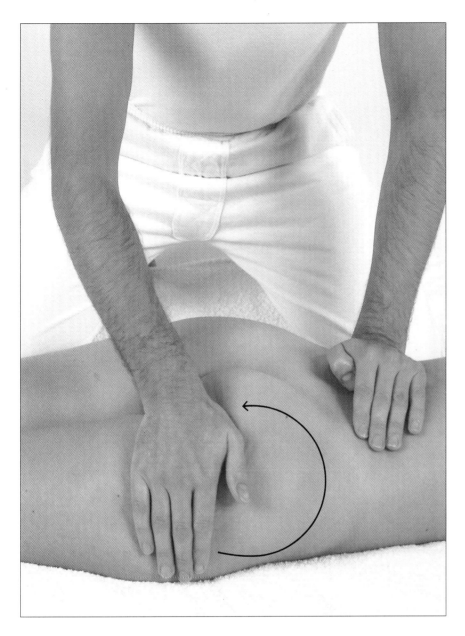

16 Rest one hand on the lower back, the other on the opposite buttock. Breathe in, and as you breathe out, lean your weight into the heel of the hand on the buttock, pushing it in and around the hip. Keep your fingers relaxed and in contact with the buttock. Continue the movement for five circles. Increase the pressure slightly each time so you build up to a pressure that is comfortable and satisfying for your partner. This stroke is a wonderful completion to the back-of-legs sequence.

Common Ailments

Before you start to massage your partner, always ask if there are any physical problems. Here is a list of the most common leg complaints you are likely to encounter and what the best course of action is in each case: whether or not a massage would help and when medical attention is advisable.

● **Calf Cramps**
These may occur for no obvious reason and can be effectively solved with effleurage and deep kneading.

Marjoram is the perfect oil to use.
● **Cellulite and Fluid Retention**
Both are eased by massage, which improves the circulation of blood and the return of lymph fluid. Long, flowing effleurage strokes assist a sluggish lymphatic system. Deep kneading and petrissage on the thighs and buttocks can help disperse fatty deposits.
● **Sciatica**
Pain is felt down the centre of the back of the thigh and the centre and

outside of the calf. Light effleurage can be very helpful here particularly with soothing camomile and lavender oils. Do not apply much pressure.
● **Varicose Veins**
These can often be prevented with the help of massage by assisting and encouraging proper circulation. Avoid petrissage, kneading or wringing strokes. Rosemary, juniper and geranium essential oils are all helpful.

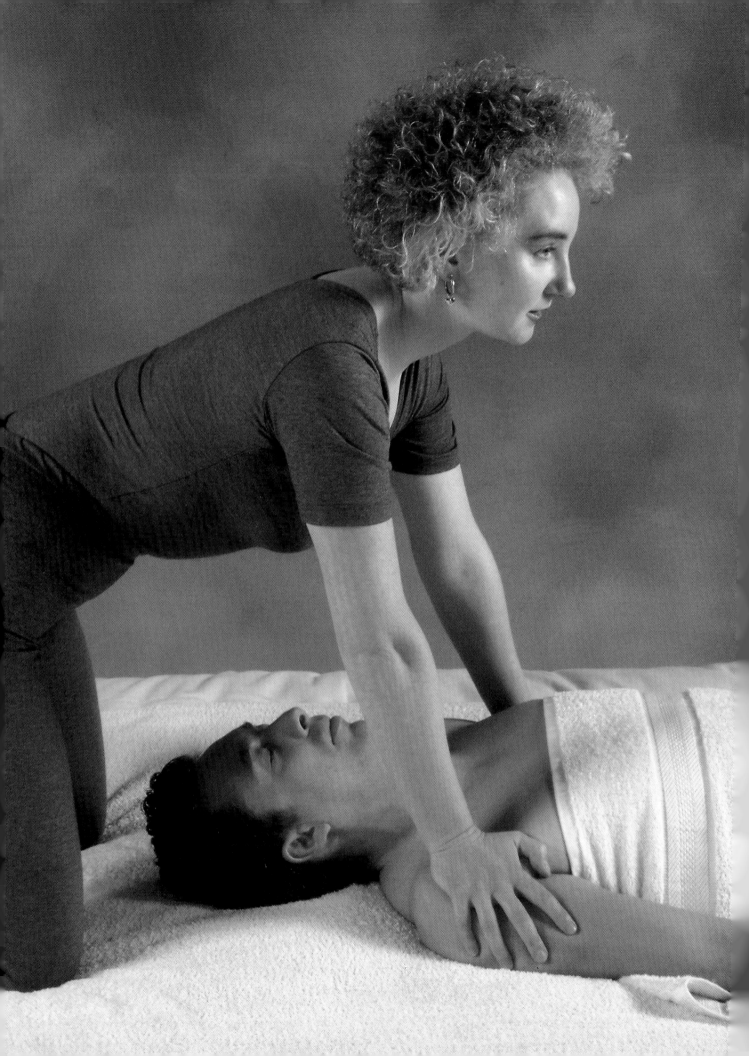

4

Chest and Neck

T he chest and neck are undoubtedly the most rewarding areas of the body to massage. Working directly on the skin here with oil can produce dramatic results in terms of relaxation. Your partner may feel as if he has had a full body treatment.

The upper chest can feel vulnerable when touched. This is because the heart and part of the lungs are housed here. Our feelings of sadness and disappointment get stored and hidden in this particular area of the body. When someone sobs heavily, the whole chest heaves. The heart is the seat of our emotions and our language reflects this connection. A person may be 'broken-hearted' with grief or find that his or her 'heart stopped' with shock. Someone unloving is often referred to as 'hard-hearted'.

The upper chest, and the heart in particular, would seem to have a need to express and receive love. When this need is unfulfilled or we deny or are denied the opportunity to express this emotion, we experience attendant physical symptoms. The shape of our body begins to reflect this emotional state. Rounded shoulders develop to protect and shield the heart area from further upset.

Reassuring massage in this area can encourage people to feel safe enough to let go of their defences. In case of emotional upset, or trauma, a sympathetic touch on the upper chest can sometimes be enough to bring grief or sadness to the surface. If this is the case, reassure your partner that this is perfectly normal and acceptable. Over a period of time, massage will help ease and soothe not only the body's armour but the emotional and mental armour as well.

The chest and neck store a great deal of our emotional tension. Massage in this area can be enormously rewarding and reassuring.

Chest and Neck

The head's position at the top of the spine is kept balanced by the co-ordinated action of the neck muscles. Looking at the chest and neck area from behind (*see bottom right*), the trapezius is the largest muscle. It is also an important component of the head-support mechanism. Problems often arise in this area if the head is held too far forward as sustained effort from the upper fibres of the trapezius is needed to support it. This can lead to neck-and-shoulder strain and headaches.

The upper-chest area is dominated by the pectoralis major muscle, lying over and attached to the upper rib-cage. This muscle's action is to pull the arms together. Tension in this area can cause rounding of the shoulders and a possible restriction to thoracic expansion, which can lead to respiratory difficulties. Many people store tension in the upper body and neck. This can partly be attributed to postural problems and to poor co-ordination of upper-limb activity. It could be that, due to a reflexive response to stress, the shoulders and neck become hunched defensively against events over which we feel we have no control. Massage has always been used to great effect to release the fatigue and tension from this vulnerable area which, if left unchecked, may have a severe debilitating effect on the physical, psychological and emotional balance of the individual.

All the lymphatic systems of the body, which carry away toxic materials and waste products from the tissues in the lymph fluid, finally drain into two ducts in the thoracic cavity. Here, the detoxified lymph fluid is returned to the circulation through veins in the upper chest. Massage in this area will therefore help this process.

Although massage can be of enormous benefit, it alone may not be sufficient to deal with certain problems in the chest and neck. Postural correction or counselling may be necessary in some cases. Remember that it is always essential to deal with the root cause of the problem, not merely the manifestation of it.

THE CHEST AND NECK MUSCLES EXPLAINED

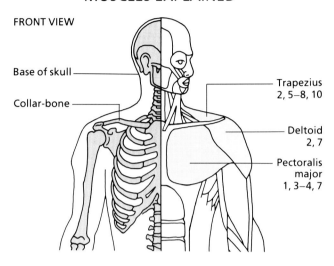

FRONT VIEW

Base of skull
Collar-bone
Trapezius 2, 5–8, 10
Deltoid 2, 7
Pectoralis major 1, 3–4, 7

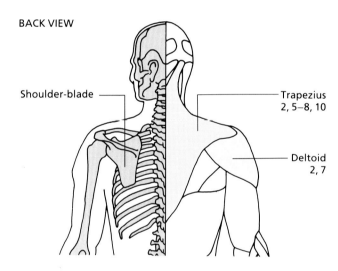

BACK VIEW

Shoulder-blade
Trapezius 2, 5–8, 10
Deltoid 2, 7

Numbers refer to steps in the following sequence, showing at which stage each muscle is worked upon.

Lying on the front of the chest wall, the pectoralis major is a broad, flat muscle connecting the rib-cage, the collar-bone and the humerus. The deltoid muscle lies on the part of the shoulder furthest from the neck and works on the arm. The trapezius is a large muscle that rises from the cervical and thoracic regions of the spine, and at its upper end from the base of the skull. All the fibres then pass out to insert into the shoulder-blade. The trapezius serves to support the head and works on the shoulders as well. Tension in this muscle can spread to other areas.

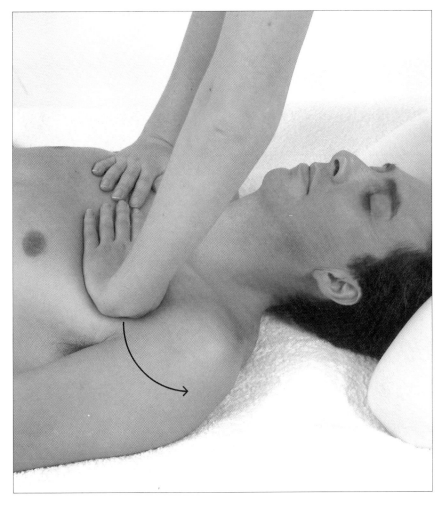

1 Begin this sequence by asking your partner to lie on his back. If your partner is a woman, protect her privacy by covering her with a towel up to the chest area. Position your knees astride your partner's head, parallel to his ears. Being too distant makes it difficult to carry out the strokes easily; too near, and your partner may feel uncomfortable. Apply the oil to your hands. Place them, slowly and gradually, on the upper chest with your fingers facing each other. Make sure that you do not lean into the chest, merely rest the hands to establish contact here. Make sure you are totally comfortable; your partner will be able to sense if you are not. Maintain contact here for at least 10 seconds. When you are ready, begin to effleurage by slowly gliding the hands away from each other towards the shoulders. The pressure here should be firm but not heavy.

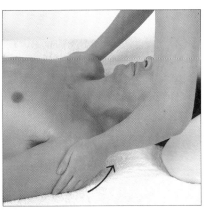

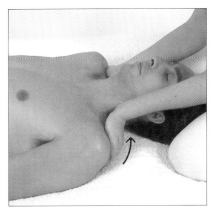

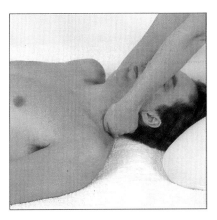

2 Maintaining your position, wrap the hands around the shoulders. Increase the pressure and push the shoulders down (*see above left*). Keep your fingers close together and relaxed. Be flexible with your body, moving forward slightly here to increase the momentum in your hands. Scoop your hands under the shoulders (*see above middle*). Bring your hands up underneath the neck

until the fingers touch. Cup the hands, one on top of the other, under the neck. Keep them well under the neck, not allowing the thumbs to slip onto the throat. Pull your hands towards you slowly, leaning back so that the neck receives a gentle stretch (*see above right*). Be careful not to let your hands come up onto the face and drag the skin or pull the ears. Draw the hands up to the base of the skull

and gently release them. Repeat the entire stroke, three to five times, beginning on the front of the chest (*see step 1*). Finish by drawing the hands up the neck and continue the stroke up the back of the head and off. Your intention here is not to lift the head but simply to continue the slow, gliding, stretching movement of your hands. Do this very slowly so your partner can fully relax his head.

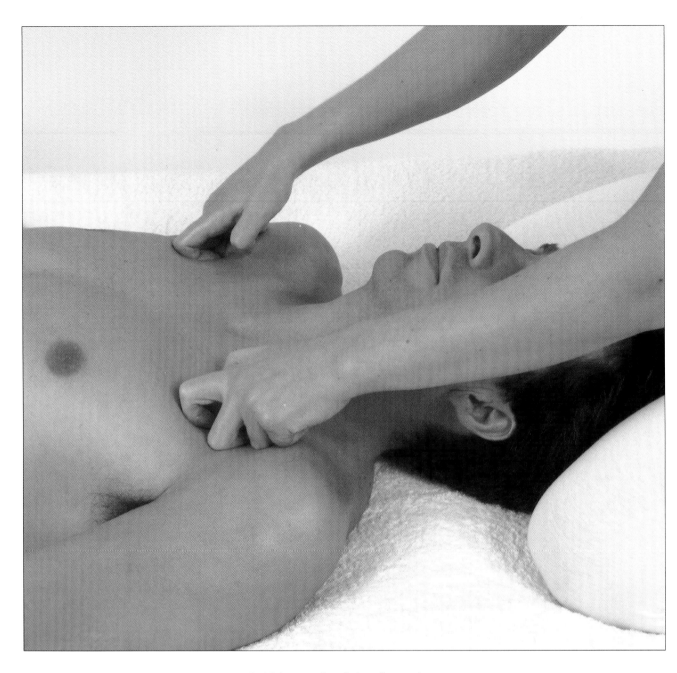

3 Make your hands into fists and place them on the upper chest, with the top section of the fingers resting on the body. Rotate the fingers around the upper chest. Move the hands all over the area, keeping them in this position and in contact with the body. Work deeper into the fleshy areas in front of the armpits. If you have trouble co-ordinating both hands, simply rest one while you work with the other. If you are working on a man with a hairy chest, be careful not to pull the hairs. This stroke also feels wonderful when extended onto the upper arms.

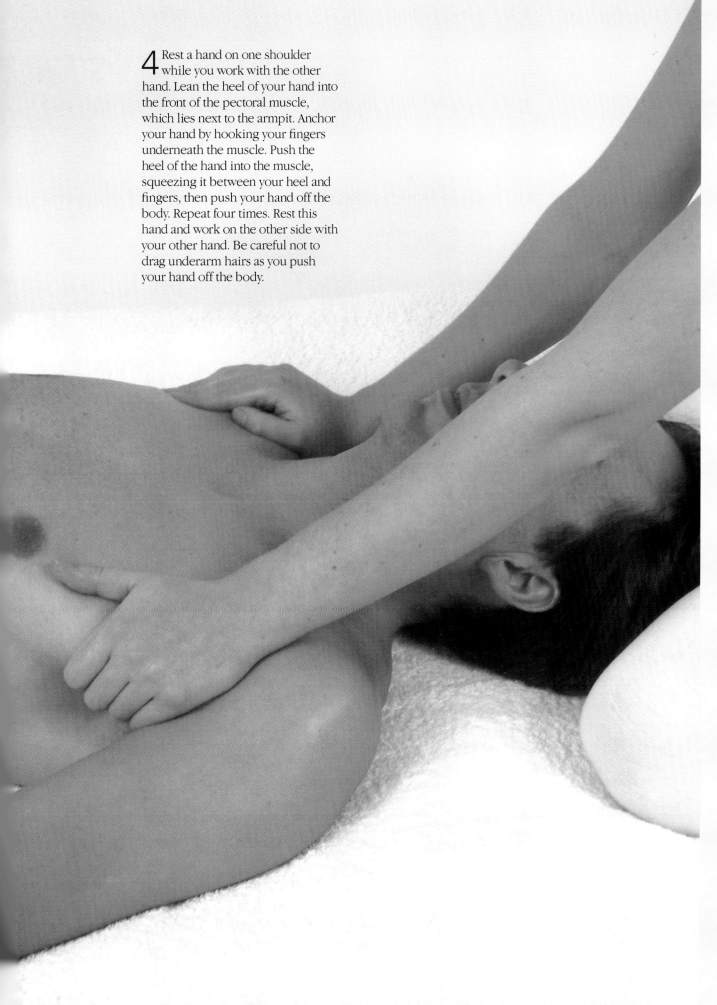

4 Rest a hand on one shoulder while you work with the other hand. Lean the heel of your hand into the front of the pectoral muscle, which lies next to the armpit. Anchor your hand by hooking your fingers underneath the muscle. Push the heel of the hand into the muscle, squeezing it between your heel and fingers, then push your hand off the body. Repeat four times. Rest this hand and work on the other side with your other hand. Be careful not to drag underarm hairs as you push your hand off the body.

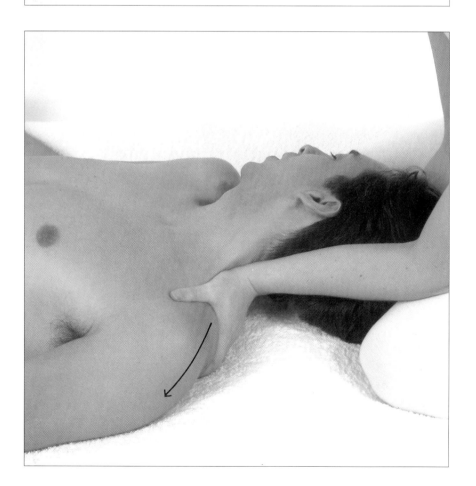

5 Using both your hands, turn your
partner's head to one side, very
gently and slowly. Allow his head to
rest on one of your hands. Lean your
other hand into the side of the neck
furthest from your partner's face and
squeeze the muscles between fingers
and thumb. Squeeze all along the
neck muscles, leaning your body
weight into your hand for extra depth.
Be careful not to let your thumb slide
onto the throat.

6 Place your hand at the top of the
neck. Push into the neck, down
and off at the shoulder. Bring your
hand straight back to the starting
position and repeat two to three
times. Avoid the throat area by
keeping your hand at the back of
the neck and under the shoulders.

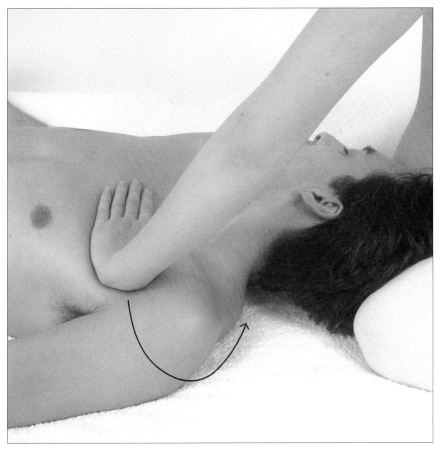

7 Keeping the head in the same position, place your hand on the chest below the collar bone (*see left*). Push into your hand and glide it across the chest, increasing the pressure as you move over the shoulder. Scoop the hand slowly around the shoulder, pushing it away from you towards the feet. Pull your hand very slowly up the neck, leaning your body back to increase the stretch (*see below*). Take care to keep the hand to the back of the neck and avoid the ear. Continue the pull right up to and off the head. Repeat the entire step from the beginning. Turn the head carefully to the other side and repeat steps 5, 6 and 7.

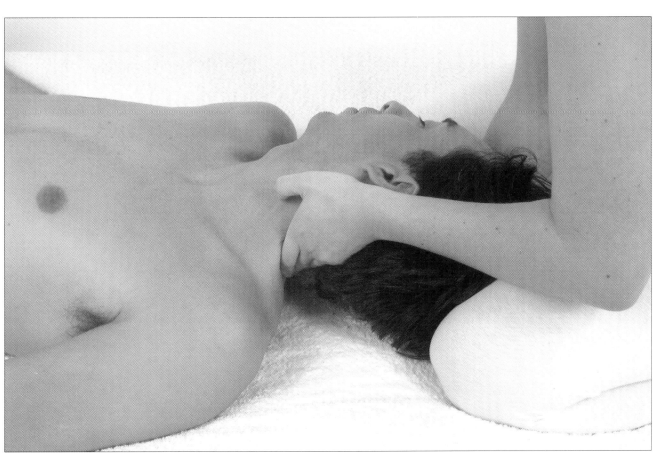

8 Bring your partner's head back to a central position very gently and slowly, using both your hands to support it fully during the movement. Rest one hand on the shoulder. Place your other hand on the opposite shoulder grasping the muscle between your hand, with your thumb on top and fingers underneath (*see right*). Lean your hand well into the muscle to get a more effective squeeze. Work thoroughly in this way all along the length of the muscle, making sure that the thumb does not slip onto the throat. When you feel that you have worked on one side of the body thoroughly, rest the hand and repeat the entire movement on the other side with the other hand.

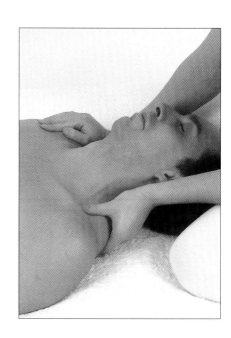

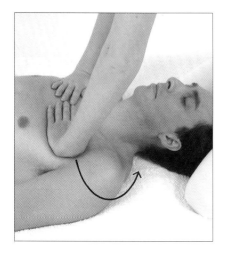

9 Place both hands on the chest. Lean in and glide the hands across the chest, under the shoulders, up the back of the neck and off at the base of the skull (*see above*).

10 Place the heel of both hands on the top of the shoulders (*see right*). Breathe in. As you breathe out, lean in to push the shoulders away from you. Push towards the feet, not down into the floor. It helps to lean forward and down, without coming up onto your knees, so you can direct your weight into the body. As a variation, push one shoulder and then the other, setting up a relaxing rhythm. If you are completing the sequence here, 'ground' your partner by moving to the feet and holding them for at least 20 seconds.

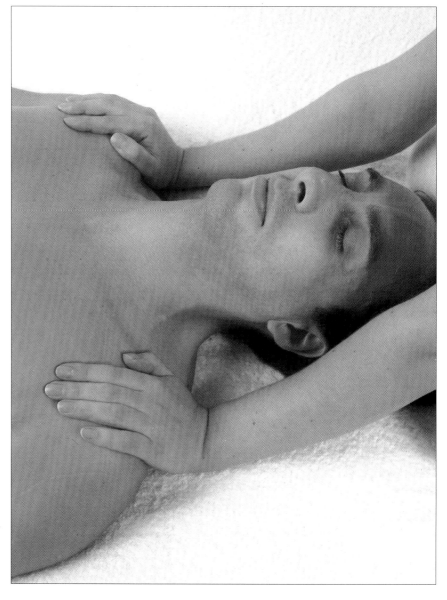

Additional Sequence

The following additional sequence is a wonderful way of completing the work in the chest and neck area. The strokes shown here serve to ease tension in the head, particularly at the base of the skull, and to loosen the scalp. Although we are familiar with the notion of tension in the body, we rarely think of our head or scalp as being stiff or tense. There is, in fact, a thin layer of muscle covering the entire skull that tightens when we are tense, causing headaches and a feeling of anxiety. By loosening this muscle and relieving tension here, a head massage will create tremendous relaxation throughout the whole body.

I have found this additional sequence to be particularly appreciated by people whose job involves a lot of 'head work', such as accountants and journalists. The work on the base of the skull is particularly good for releasing pent-up tension. It can have an enormously liberating effect. This sequence can be added on at the end of the chest and neck sequence.

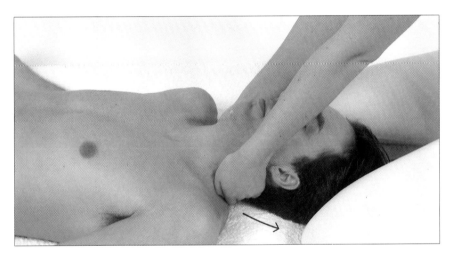

1 Apply the oil to your hands if necessary. Place your hands below the collar-bone, fingers facing each other. Lean in and slowly sweep around the shoulders, bringing your hands to meet under the neck. Cup your hands together, one on top of the other. Pull your hands slowly towards you. Bring them right up onto the head in this cupped position for the next stroke.

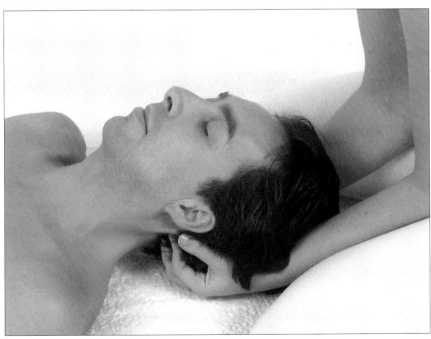

2 Separate your hands and position your fingertips under the head, on the ridge along the base of the skull. Make sure that they are not merely on the head itself or the neck. Cradle the head comfortably in the rest of your hands. Let your fingers rest then press here for at least 20 seconds. Then, very slowly, rotate the fingers in tiny circles. If your fingers cannot reach the entire area, move your hands to enable them to do so.

3 Bring your hands up onto the head. Press your fingertips into the sides of your partner's head. Rotate your fingers slowly all over the head. Make sure you are pressing deeply enough to move the scalp and loosen the tension. You can vary this movement by resting one hand and working with the other. Concentrate on the areas around the ears and immediately above the forehead. Begin the movement very slowly, increasing the pace only gradually. For a more stimulating effect, work the fingertips vigorously on the scalp, but only if you can maintain the depth of your pressure meanwhile. This will probably take you some time to master fully.

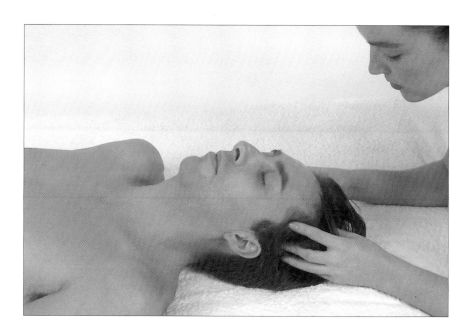

4 Lift your hands and position them with the fingers pointing downwards and palms facing you. Draw the hands slowly through the hair towards you. If your partner has long hair, try to include the entire length of the hair. Concentrate this movement on the centre of the head and then each side in turn. Think about drawing out all the unnecessary thoughts and concerns that your partner is holding in his head. This is a most exquisite movement and works wonderfully with the previous step. Together they will leave your partner's head feeling lighter and cleaner. The next step completes this relaxing sequence.

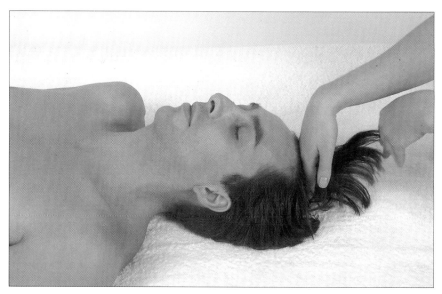

5 With your thumb and forefinger, gently tug a small tuft of hair on the hair-line. Hold the hair and pull firmly so that the forehead moves. Do this rhythmically, pulling first on one side and then the other. Work only on the hair-line. This movement is tremendous for releasing tension and worry lines in the forehead.

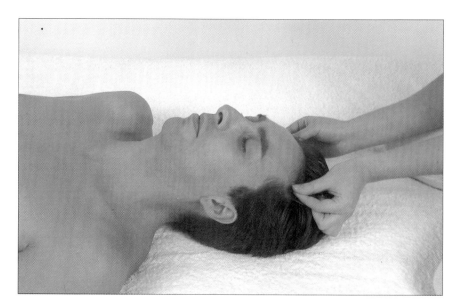

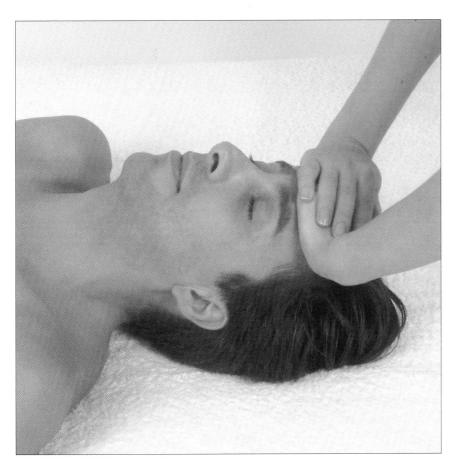

6 Bring your hands to the forehead very gradually, resting one and placing the other on top. Make sure that you are relaxed or your hands will not be completely still and calming. If you need to, change your position so you are sitting on a cushion rather than kneeling. Stay here for at least 20 seconds. By now your partner should be feeling extremely tranquil and relaxed. Bring your hands off, very slowly, one at a time. Encourage him to stay still and remain lying down for a few minutes. If you are just doing this sequence and not proceeding to work elsewhere on the body, move to your partner's feet. Simply hold them for 20 seconds to 'ground' your partner.

Common Ailments

Before you start to massage your partner, always ask if there are any physical problems. The following is a list of the most common chest and neck complaints you are likely to come across. It tells you what the best course of action is in each case: whether or not a massage would help and when medical attention is advisable.

● **Aching pectoral muscles**
Over-zealous weight-training can often lead to this complaint. Kneading the pectorals will be particularly useful here. Your partner will let you know how much pressure is required. If these muscles are being developed more than those of the back, this would be creating long-term postural habits and chronic tension problems. Good oils to use here are marjoram and lavender.

● **Asthma**
This condition, like bronchitis and emphysema, affects the upper chest and makes breathing difficult for the sufferer. All three cause rounded shoulders and tight pectoral muscles. The sufferer will tend to breathe shallowly, only from the upper-chest cavity. This should not be encouraged by working deeply on the upper chest. The best thing to do here is to relax the area with gentle effleurage and release the pectoral muscles with mild kneading. Keep the pressure very light. Avoid leaning your body weight into the shoulders. Frankincense or lavender are good oils to use in this area.

● **Cardiac rehabilitation**
If your partner is in the recovery period following heart surgery, massage must be attempted only if

you have the permission of the medical consultant. After such an operation your partner is likely to feel worried and tense. So, the calming and relaxing effects of massage can be enormously helpful here. Gentle, rhythmic effleurage is best. It will lower blood pressure and help your partner to sleep. Use a gentle oil like neroli.

● **Wry Neck**
This is a condition where the head is pulled down and rotated to one side, leading to a physical shortening of the tissues. Someone with this condition would be under the care of a medical expert. Massage would be very helpful here, however, as there are no specific contra-indications that suggest massage could be harmful. Lavender, grapefruit and geranium are useful oils.

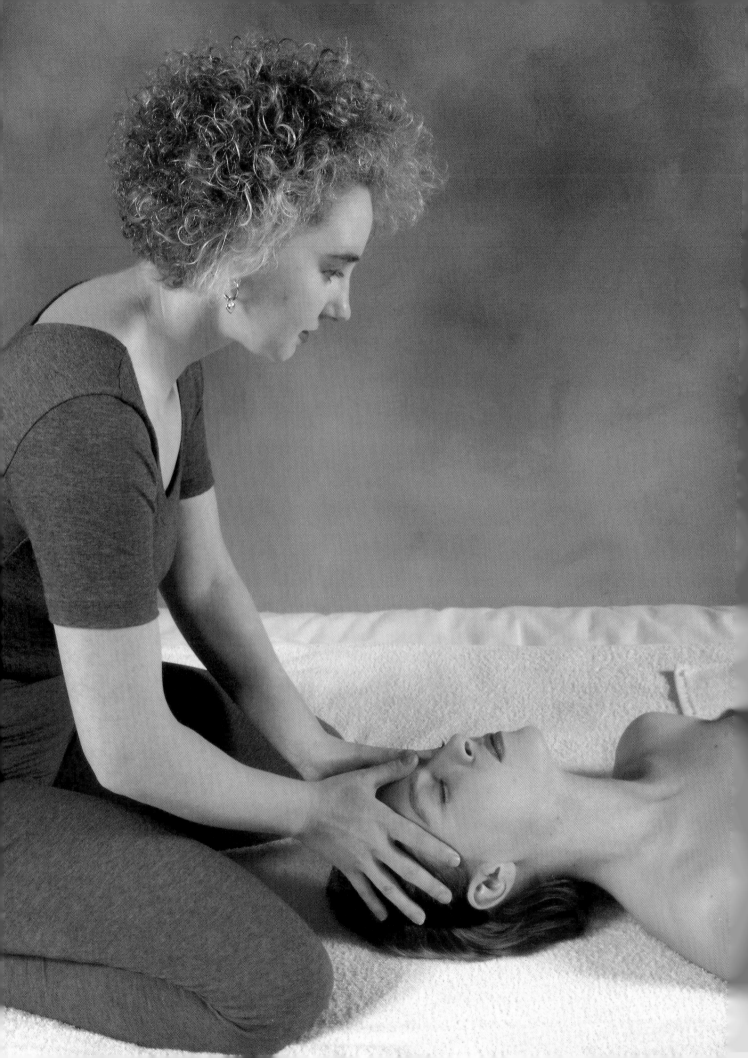

5

Face and Head

The face is the most exposed area of the body, revealing our thoughts and feelings to the world. When we block our true feelings and express those that are more acceptable, this conflict will register as tension in the facial muscles. The phrase 'grin and bear it' describes such a situation perfectly. Chronic tension and conflict can shape the face into a permanent expression. This is especially noticeable in older faces. A person's whole life or, more accurately, his or her conclusions about it, are clearly etched in the contours of the face. A lifetime of resignation or disappointment shows in collapsed muscles, a tired expression and a lifeless pallor.

Tense facial muscles are a primary cause of premature ageing. The muscles underlying the skin give the face its shape and contour. As they contract they cause the skin to wrinkle giving us our expression lines. If the muscles remain tense and do not relax they lead to permanent wrinkles. The most noticeable and immediate improvement you will see through massage is in the relief of a furrowed brow. All the forehead strokes will help to smooth out the frown lines and worried expression. These strokes also indirectly soothe the brain through the nerve channels beneath the forehead.

The head is another area, that, like the face, we do not think of as holding tension. There is a layer of muscle covering the skull, however, which tightens when we are tense and causes headaches. People with mentally taxing careers are prone to such tension. Massage can loosen it, leaving your partner feeling clear-headed and looking years younger.

The face and head are often the most overworked parts of the body. Massage here releases stress from the entire body and produces a deeply relaxed and refreshed outlook.

Face and Head

The face is a relatively small area that contains many intricate muscles. The muscles here do not attach bone to bone as is the case with the rest of the body, but facial bones to skin and areas of skin to other parts of the face. This allows for our variety of facial expressions.

The jaw is an exception. It articulates with the skull at the temporo-mandibular joint just in front of the ear to allow speech and chewing. This is often a site of tension, particularly for people who grip their jaw or grind their teeth at night. The muscle most affected here is the masseter, which is often referred to as the 'chewing' muscle.

The lips are surrounded by the orbicularis oris and the levator anguli muscles, which lift the corners of the mouth. Surrounding the eye is the orbicularis oculi muscle, while on the forehead lies the temporalis muscle. Facial tension is brought about through movements such as frowning, screwing up the eyes and clenching the jaw. Massage on the face helps to release this tension, which, if left unchecked, will keep the muscles in a steady state of contraction, causing headaches and the formation of permanent wrinkles and furrows on the forehead. Massage can relax taut muscles and tone up those that are underused and have shrivelled up as a result, making the skin sag, usually around the jaw.

The head provides a constant supply of blood to the brain. Massage on the head helps this flow and prevents congestion. Headaches can be experienced on most parts of the head. A common site is the frontal area, across the forehead. The pain may also be felt on the sides of the head, the temporal area, or at the top of the head, the parietal area. People with constitutional weakness, who may suffer from poor circulation or a hardening of the arteries, are prone to parietal headaches. The occipital area, the base of the skull, is also a prime site for headaches. This is commonly caused by tension in the trapezius muscle, obstructing blood flow and causing congestion.

THE FACE AND HEAD MUSCLES EXPLAINED

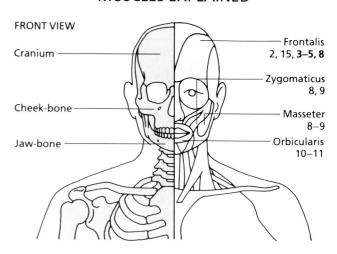

FRONT VIEW

Cranium

Cheek-bone

Jaw-bone

Frontalis
2, 15, **3–5, 8**

Zygomaticus
8, 9

Masseter
8–9

Orbicularis
10–11

Numbers refer to steps in the following sequence, showing at which stage each muscle is worked upon. Numbers in bold type apply to the second sequence.

The face is the most intricate area of the body to massage due to its small size and great number of muscles. The frontalis, zygomaticus and orbicularis muscles are concerned with producing facial expressions. The masseter is one of a group of muscles that moves the jaw-bone up and down during chewing. The cheek-bone is the ridge that can be felt just below the eyes. Several facial muscles attach to it. The cranium comprises the bones of the skull.

The sinuses are hollow cavities in the skull lined with mucous membrane. These cavities serve to make the skull lighter and also provide resonance for the voice. They are mainly found in the frontal part of the head and down either side of the nose. The lining of these sinuses can become swollen and inflamed if infected material comes into contact with them. Due to the enclosed nature of the sinuses, this can be extremely painful. The maxillary sinuses, in particular, can become infected through taking in dirty water during swimming. Massaging the forehead will help to stimulate lymphatic drainage and may help to assuage the debilitating pain of chronic sinusitis.

Face

The face is the smallest and most sensitive area of the body you will work on. It requires you to use your hands with greater dexterity and precision than you have done in previous massage routines in this course. A good facial massage can greatly improve the skin's health and appearance. It boosts the circulation and lymph flow, clearing away toxins and making for a glowing complexion.

The movements on the cheeks involve using only your fingertips with very light pressure. You will need to be particularly sensitive in your use of pressure everywhere on the face. The amount you use will vary enormously between one person and the next. Do not hesitate to check what feels best for your partner.

You will find that people, particularly women, are generally anxious to avoid having the skin dragged, fearing that this might slacken the skin or contribute to a loss of elasticity. It is therefore important to guard against pulling the skin in your movements, particularly with the rotation on the cheeks and the gliding strokes above and below the lips.

Remember to check whether your partner is wearing make-up so that you can avoid smudging it. She may ask you to use her favourite moisturising lotion instead of an oil, or to use no lubrication at all. Not everyone will appreciate getting oil on their hair, so you may need to dry your hands before moving on from the face to work on the scalp.

It is important to be able to lean into the strokes on the forehead so a kneeling position is essential. If you need to, change to a sitting position for all the other strokes. A soft pillow under the neck and head will make your partner very comfortable. Leave plenty of time for your partner to rest after this treatment, as it tends to have a quite soporific effect.

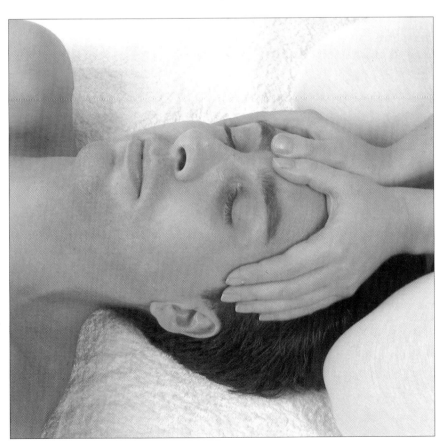

1 Kneel astride your partner's head. If your hands are dry, apply half a teaspoon of oil to your hands. Bring your hands to rest on the forehead very gradually and deliberately. Position the thumbs and the heels of your hands in the centre of the forehead and wrap your fingers around the sides. Maintain a firm pressure without actually pressing into your hands. Be careful not to push the forehead down towards the eyebrows. Stay here for at least 20 seconds.

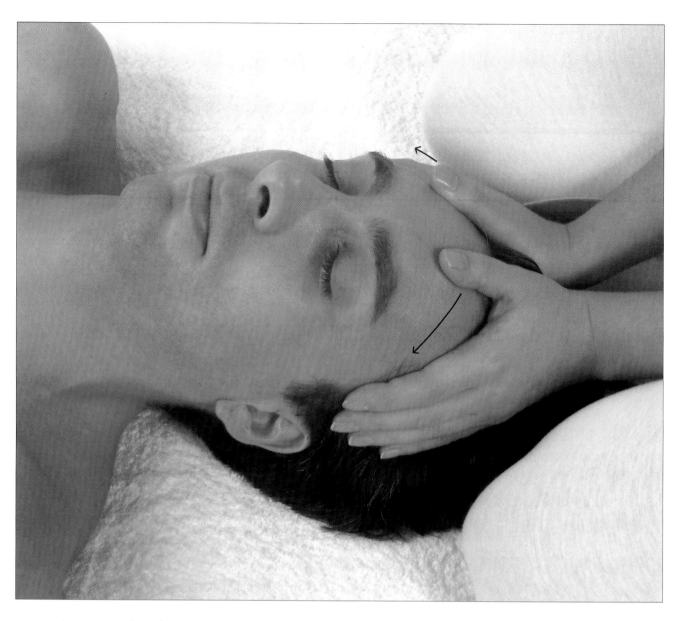

2 Breathe in. As you breathe out, lean forward slightly to transfer your weight into your thumbs and glide them across the forehead towards the ears (*see above*). Keep the thumbs relaxed but straight, with even pressure along their entire length. When you reach the ears, bring your hands back to the forehead, placing them slightly above your original position and repeat the movement. Move upwards and repeat in this way until you reach the hair-line (*see right*). Remember always to work towards the ears. Ask your partner how much pressure is comfortable. Deep pressure may feel profoundly relaxing to some but quite uncomfortable to others.

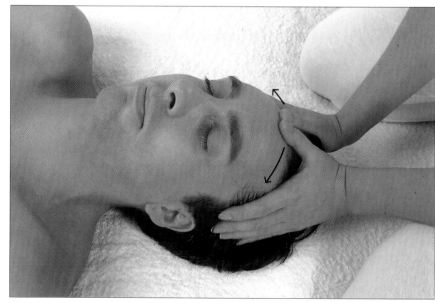

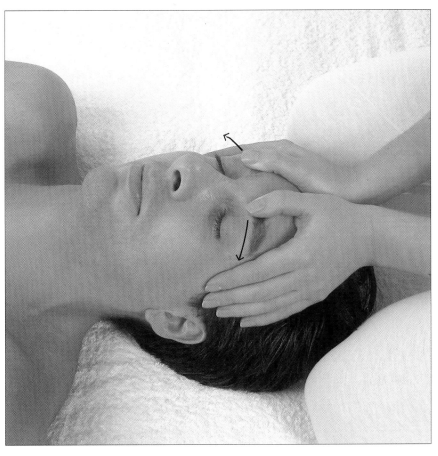

3 Lift the hands off the hair-line to rest them on the forehead, thumbs placed directly on the eyebrows. Breathe in. As you breathe out, lean forward to transfer weight into your thumbs. Draw them slowly across the eyebrows down to the ears. Then lift off the hands, return to your starting position and repeat. You can usually apply the same amount of pressure here as on the forehead, but check what is comfortable for your partner. Conclude this step by keeping your thumbs resting on the temples.

4 Press your thumbs into the temples and rotate very slowly in a clockwise direction. Check with your partner that the pressure is right. Continue rotating for at least ten circles on each side. Keep the movement very slow: the slower it is, the more relaxing and effective it will be. As a variation, simply apply the same, constant pressure with your thumbs into the temples, without rotating, for at least 20 seconds.

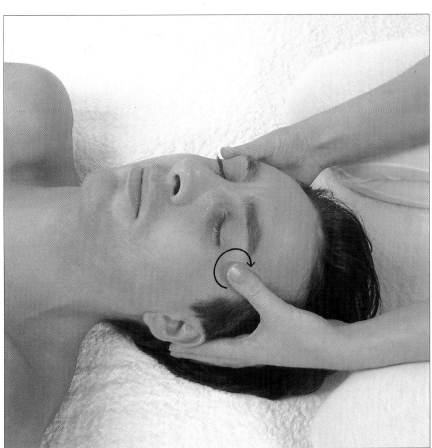

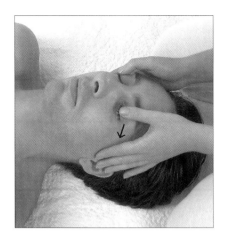

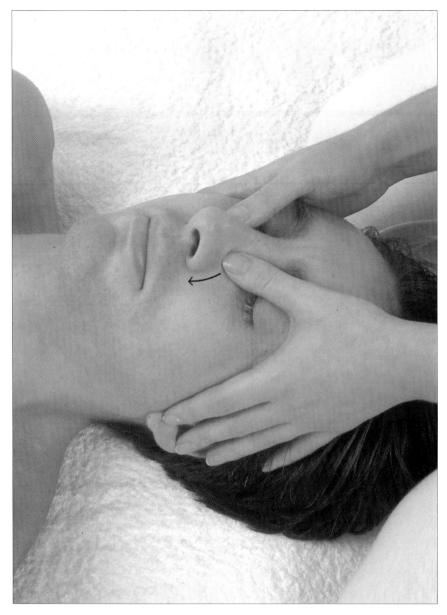

5 Making sure that your partner's eyes are closed, bring your thumbs to the inner corners of the eyes, next to the nose (*see above*). Keep your thumbs relaxed and straight. Very lightly, with no pressure whatsoever, glide your thumbs slowly across the eyelids. Continue the movement down to the ears. Lift your hands, return to your original position and repeat. It is extremely important that you do not drag the skin in this delicate area, so make sure that your touch is sufficiently gentle to glide without pulling.

6 Place your thumbs on either side of the top of the nose (*see right*). Keep the rest of your hands relaxed and in contact with the face to anchor the thumbs. Glide them slowly down the sides of the nose to the nostrils. Keep the pressure light so that you do not close the nose and inhibit breathing. Repeat. When you reach the nostrils this time, keep your thumbs there for the next stroke.

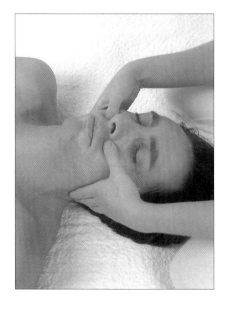

7 Keeping your thumbs in position at the base of the nose, turn your hands so that the fingers are anchored at the back of the neck (*see left*). Press your thumbs into the face just at the outside of each nostril. Apply the pressure gradually and only to a depth that your partner is comfortable with. Hold this position for 10 seconds. Do not repeat unless your partner is troubled with sinus congestion. This point is extremely useful in such cases, and this step should be repeated three times.

8 Place the pads of your three middle fingers on the cheek-bones (*see right*). Press in slightly and very slowly rotate in a small circle. Lift the fingers just enough to move onto the next section of cheek-bone. Aim to divide the area roughly into three segments, finishing near the ears. Keep the pressure light unless your partner is suffering from a head cold or sinus congestion, in which case repeat the movement three times. Rotate the fingers as deeply as your partner is comfortable with.

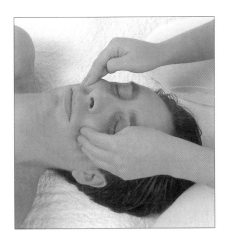

9 Continuing from step 8, without lifting your fingers away, place the pads of your three middle fingers on the face next to the ears, just below your finishing position on the cheek-bones in the previous step (*see below*). Lean your fingers in slightly and rotate them slowly, three times. Your are aiming to relieve tension in this area by rotating into the jaw socket. This stroke is particularly useful for people who grind their teeth at night and hold tension in their jaws.

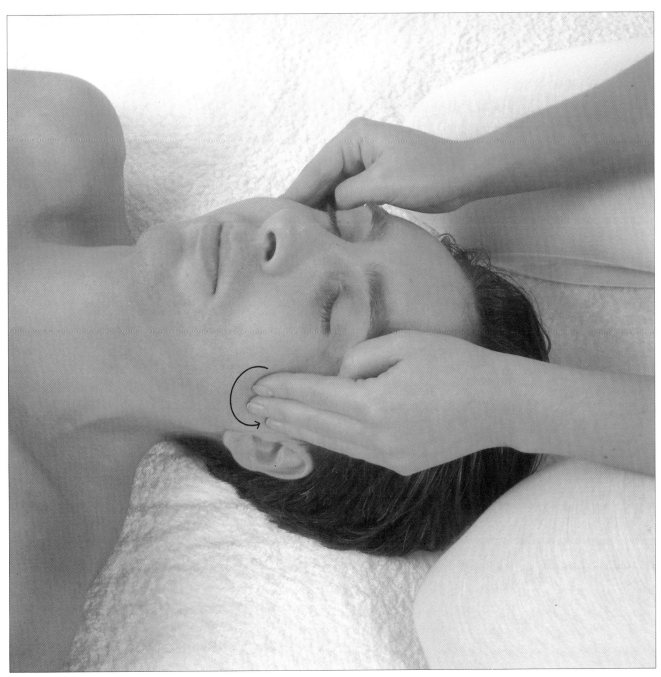

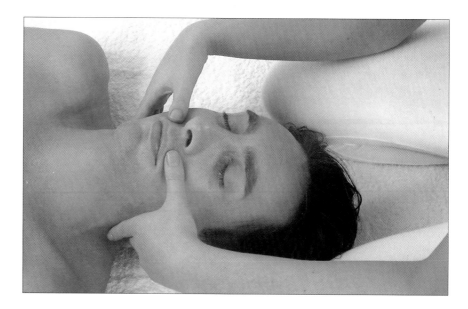

10 Wrap your hands around your partner's head to position your thumbs on the ridge between the upper lip and nose. Lean your thumbs in slightly and glide them outwards to just beyond the edge of the upper lip, maintaining the pressure. Avoid dragging the skin and glide in a straight line rather than down towards the lips. Repeat the movement twice.

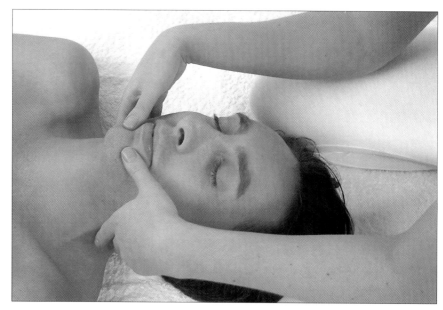

11 Move the hands down to position the thumbs along the ridge between the lower lip and chin. Lean your thumbs in with slightly more pressure than you used in the previous step. Glide across the ridge in a straight line to just beyond the edge of the lower lip, keeping your pressure constant. Repeat this movement twice. To add variety to this step, lean your thumbs in, hold for 5 seconds, then lift them off and move along the ridge. Continue in this way until you have covered the area you would have glided over.

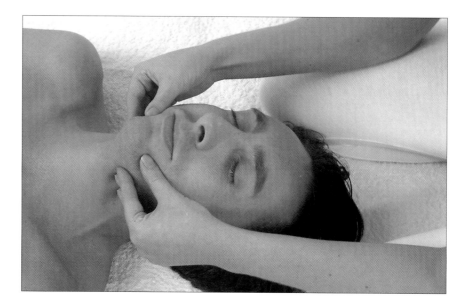

12 Hook your fingers underneath the jaw, making sure they are not touching the throat. Secure them by placing your thumbs directly below the middle of the lips. Grasp the jaw firmly but without causing discomfort to your partner. Squeeze the fingers and thumbs together into the jaw. As you press in, slowly rotate your thumbs in small circles. Keeping your hands firmly in place, move them outwards slightly, along the jaw, to repeat the rotation movement. Continue this stroke until you have reached the ears. Do not repeat unless your partner has a very tight or painful jaw. In such cases, repeat this movement twice.

13 Smoothly bring your hands from the jaw to the ears, placing your thumb and index finger on the ear-lobe (*see below*). Squeeze the ear-lobe firmly, asking your partner how much pressure is comfortable. Rotate your thumbs slowly and continue the movement upwards to include the entire ear. This stroke should feel surprisingly pleasant for your partner.

14 Cover both ears with your hands, wrapping your fingers underneath them and placing the heels of your hands on top (*see right*). Very slowly draw the hands down and off the ears. Do not pull the ears to the point of stretching them as this may feel uncomfortable. Remember to ask your partner how much pressure feels comfortable. Repeat the movement once.

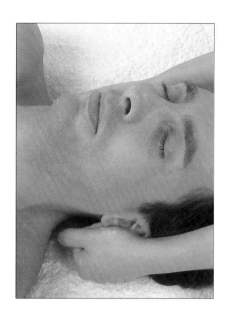

15 Rest one hand on the forehead, placing the other on top, (*see below*). Lean in to apply slight pressure. Slowly release the pressure and draw the hands back towards you. Repeat as soon as both hands are off the forehead. Then 'ground' your partner by moving to the feet and holding them for 20 seconds.

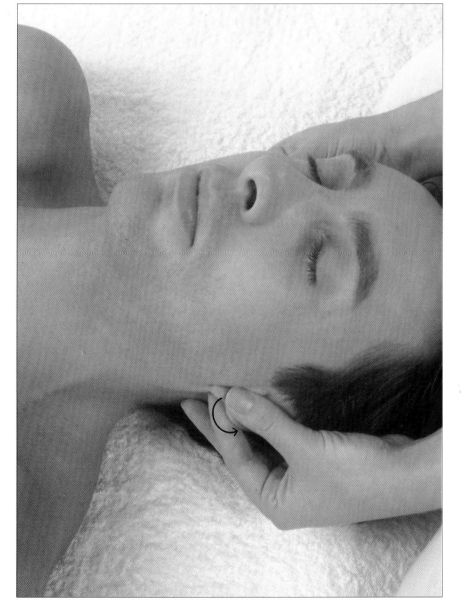

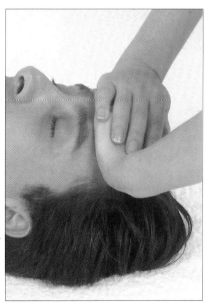

Head

The following head sequence feels wonderfully luxurious and completes the previous face treatment well. If you wish to continue straight on to the head, omit the last stroke in the face sequence (*see step 15, page 99*).

This sequence can also be carried out on its own and forms an ideal short treatment. It can take as little as 5 minutes to complete it thoroughly without any rush. The movements make contact with the entire head, including relaxing pressure on the forehead and an invigorating rub on the scalp.

Your partner might benefit from a soft pillow under the neck and head during this sequence. It is useful to ask your partner if she minds oil on her face or hair. Overlooking such details could ruin your partner's enjoyment of this treatment.

Your position can be the same as in the face sequence, kneeling behind the head. Or you could experiment with a comfortable sitting position, supporting yourself with a cushion. If you have no oil on your hands and your partner's skin is dry, use half a teaspoon of oil.

If you are not working anywhere else on the body, then I recommend you conclude by moving to the feet and holding them firmly for 30 seconds. This will help your partner feel more balanced and 'grounded'.

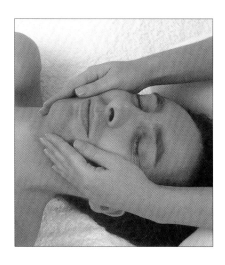

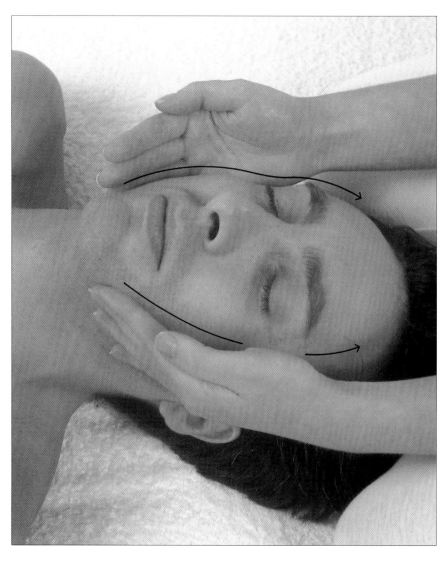

1 Place your hands around the sides of the face, lightly resting on the cheeks (*see above*). Stay here, with no pressure, for 10 seconds. Keep your hands still and calm. Check that you are relaxed and breathing comfortably, as any tension will transmit itself to your partner's face and be very noticeable.

2 Slowly draw the hands back towards you, up the sides of the face (*see right*). Keep your hands at an angle to the face so that only the edge is making contact. Continue the movement, bringing your hands up onto the forehead, resting the thumbs in the centre.

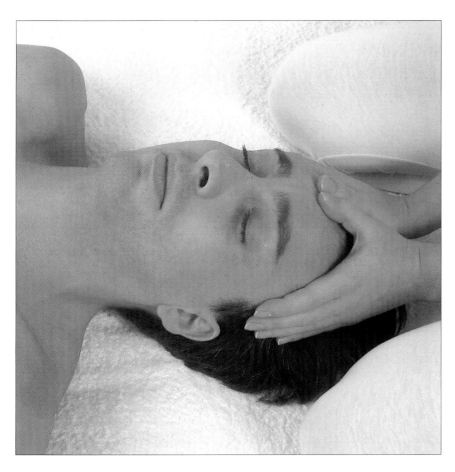

3 Make sure that your thumbs are positioned alongside each other, resting in between the eyebrows, and that your hands are relaxed and comfortably anchored on the sides of the head. Breathe in. As you breathe out, lean your body forward to drop your weight into your thumbs. Slowly draw the thumbs back towards the hair-line (*see left*), keeping your thumbs parallel to each other. You should be able to use quite deep pressure here, but quietly check with your partner what feels best. Leave your thumbs at the hair-line with your hands anchored firmly on the head.

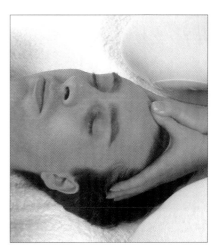

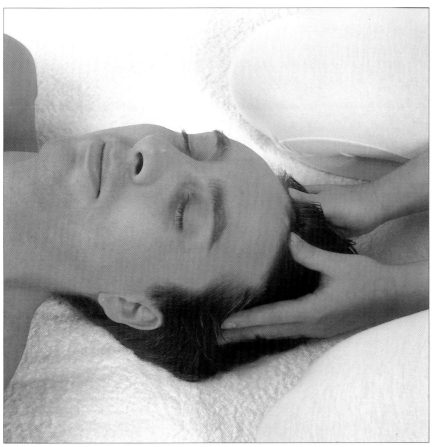

4 Place one thumb on top of the other (*see above*). Breathe in. As you breathe out, lean forward, apply pressure to the head and hold for 5 seconds. Release the thumbs and repeat the movement continually down the head as far as you can reach. It may help to imagine a line running down the centre of the head.

5 Bring your thumbs to rest either side of the line you have just worked on (*see left*). Breathe in. As you breathe out lean into your thumbs. Bring them off briefly to reposition them. Continue to apply the pressure like this down the head as far as you can reach.

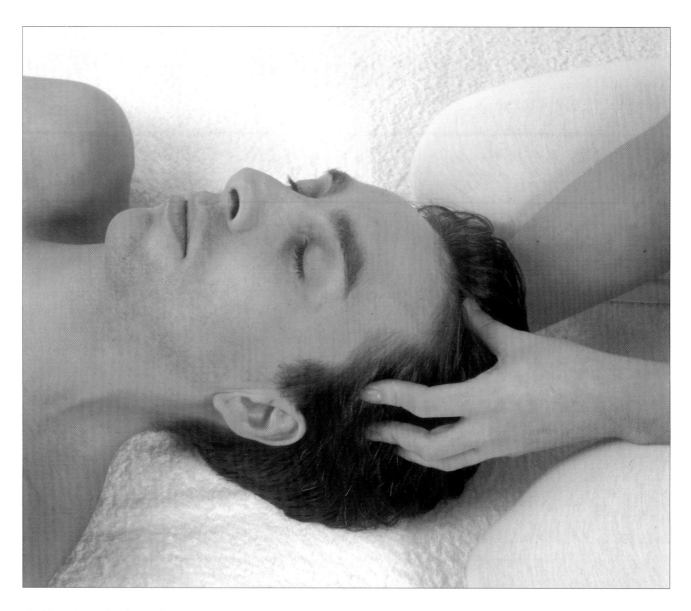

6 Place the pads of your fingers on the head (*see above*). Press into the scalp and rotate your fingers vigorously. If you find it difficult to maintain a rhythm with both hands then work with one at a time resting the other on the head. Work thoroughly all over the head, paying special attention to the area at the base of the skull.

7 Place one hand on the head, with the back of the hand upright facing the forehead. Draw the fingers slowly through the hair (*see right*) and repeat immediately with your other hand. Keep the movement flowing and continuous, both hands working in tandem. Work thoroughly on the entire head.

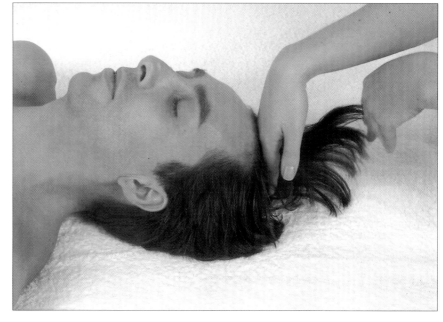

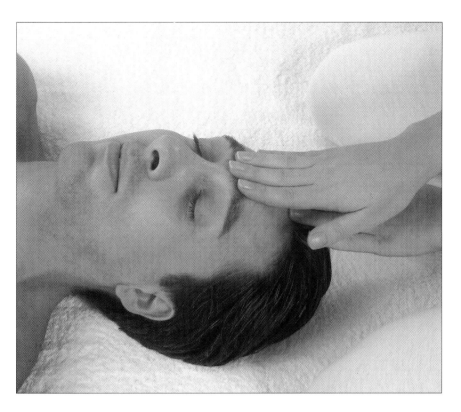

8 Slowly bring one hand to rest on the head. Place your other hand on top. Begin gradually to lean your weight into your hands and the forehead. When you have reached a comfortable depth of pressure, maintain it for at least 10 seconds. Release the pressure very slowly, so that your partner hardly notices what you are doing. Take the top hand off very gradually, followed by the other hand. As a guideline, this entire movement should take at least 30 seconds. If you are finishing your massage here, remember to ground you partner by holding the feet for 20 seconds. Then encourage him to rest for a while before getting up.

Common Ailments

Before you start to massage your partner, always ask if there are any physical problems. Here is a list of the most common face and head complaints you are likely to encounter and the best course of action in each case: whether or not a massage would help and when medical attention is advisable.

● **Headache**
This is undoubtedly the most common complaint associated with the face and head. Eyestrain, overeating, blocked sinuses and muscle tension can all cause headaches. Massage is of tremendous benefit here. Below are the four main sites of headaches and the corresponding massage treatment. All these approaches can also be applied to a migraine headache, initially concentrating the pressure specifically on the painful area. It is also helpful to use one drop of peppermint oil and three of lavender to a teaspoon of carrier oil.

Base of the skull
Rest the base of the skull on your upturned fingertips. Maintain pressure for 30 seconds. Then rotate the pads of your fingers slowly and deeply, concentrating on the problem area.

Forehead
A headache here usually benefits from very deep pressure. Begin with step 1 (see page 93) then carry out all the movements for the forehead.

Temples
Use the thumb-circling movement (see step 4, page 95). Begin with pressure for 30 seconds, taking care to apply and release it gradually.

Top of the head
Carry out the entire head sequence repeating each of the thumb-pressure strokes four times (see steps 3, 4 and 5, page 101).

● **Neuralgia**
This is a blanket term for a pain of unknown origin, possibly caused by the effect of a virus on a nerve through injury. It results in a lingering pain on the nerves of the face. Sufferers should consult a doctor. Only work here if the doctor has given permission.

● **Sinusitis**
Inflamed sinuses lead to pain in the head and face. Massage can be very effective here. Concentrate on the gliding strokes down the nose and across the cheeks (see steps 2–6, pages 94–96, steps 10 and 11, page 98). Repeat them five times. Apply pressure to the point at the edge of the nostrils five times (see step 7, page 96), holding for 10 seconds each time. Use two drops of rosemary oil in your vegetable oil during the sequence.

● **Stroke**
An interruption of the blood supply to one half of the body leaves the muscle contracted and taut. Massage can help a lot here, depending on severity. A blend of one drop of lavender oil and two of neroli in your vegetable oil is excellent for use here.

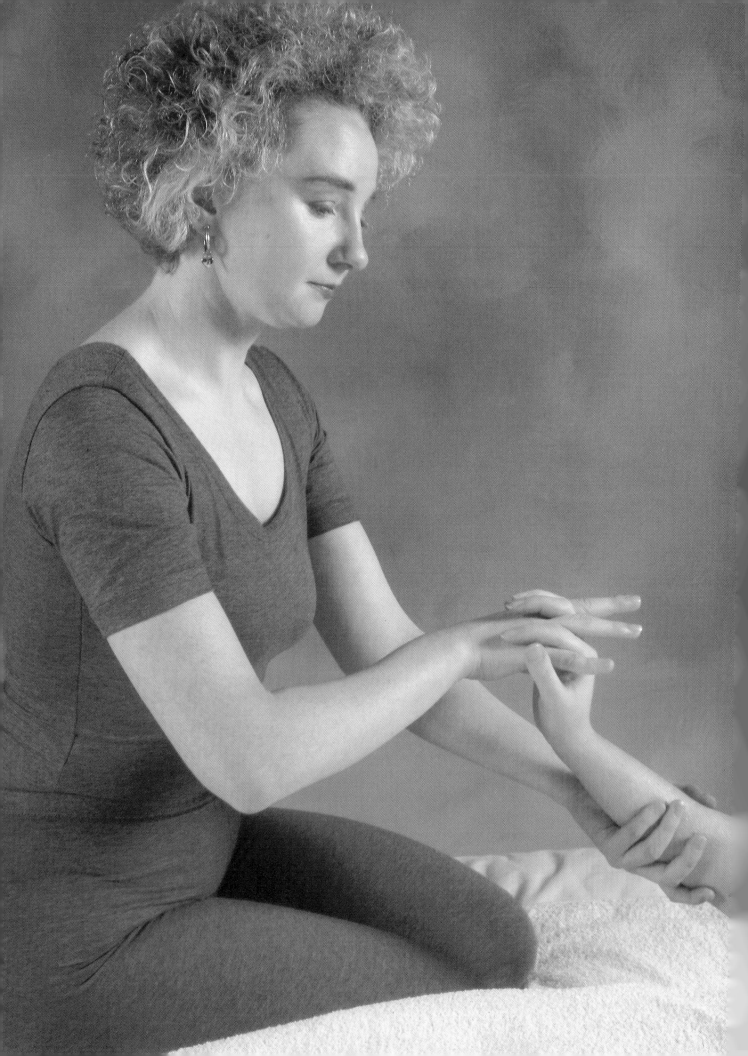

6

Arms and Hands

We use our arms and hands to interact with our environment and to communicate our feelings. They can express our emotions – from embracing a loved one to hitting out in rage. Our language is full of expressions that describe how we handle the world through our arms, such as 'getting to grips with things' and 'getting our hands dirty'.

The extent to which we express and fulfil ourselves in our lives is revealed in our arms. People who hold their arms close to the body, whether standing or lying down, will be uneasy about taking up much space or asserting themselves. Their arms will appear weak and lifeless and they will experience themselves as powerless and victimized. Feelings and longings will be buried in the belly and shoulders, unable to find expression through the arms and hands.

Our hands, likewise, reveal much of ourselves that we do not express openly. Modern documentary makers understand this well. Witness the subject speaking calmly while the camera focuses on their wringing hands, exposing their inner turmoil. It is healthy to use our hands to express ourselves. Studies in the UK have shown how elderly people who cuddle and stroke a loved pet enjoy a much better morale and lower blood pressure than others.

The purpose and potential of a good, sympathetic arms and hands treatment is to give the suppressed individual permission to expand and take up more space. Furthermore, all of us can benefit from being more in touch with our arms and hands to express hidden or unspoken communication.

*Massage helps to release tension and
blocked emotions from the shoulder, chest
and throat region and, invigorates
tired, lifeless arms.*

Arms and Hands

The muscles and joints of the shoulder allow great freedom and variety of movement in this area. The muscles here stabilize the shoulder girdle to allow manipulative work to be performed by the arm and hand. People often experience tension in these muscles. This is usually caused by excessively stressful physical activity.

The deltoid muscle gives the shoulder its rounded appearance and prevents downward movement of the arm. The flat pectoralis major muscle at the front of the body works to pull the arm across the chest. At the back of the body, the trapezius muscle acts on the shoulder-blade whilst the latissimus dorsi muscle passes into the upper arm.

On the upper arm lies the biceps muscle. People engaged in heavy manual activity may strain this muscle. The triceps muscle is also found on the upper arm. It is used to a great extent in movements such as pushing or lifting a weight above the head. Weight trainers who overdevelop the biceps often produce painful tension, potentially resulting in a shortening of the muscle. If the pectorals are similarly over-developed, this can encourage a rounding of the shoulders. In extreme cases, restricted movement may also be a feature.

At the elbow, the radius bone moves around the ulna bone, allowing the forearm to rotate in movements such as pouring. The flexor muscles of the forearm allow us to grip. Activities that involve gripping, such as rowing, racquet sports or even carrying shopping, will affect these forearm muscles. Releasing tension here through massage can reduce shortening of the muscles and release tension from the hands.

The wrist is a small area full of tendons, nerves and blood vessels. This lack of space and density of activity here means that any inflammation or bruising can be devastating, made worse by the lack of muscle to protect the area. Injuries to the hand can, therefore, be very serious indeed.

THE ARMS MUSCLES EXPLAINED

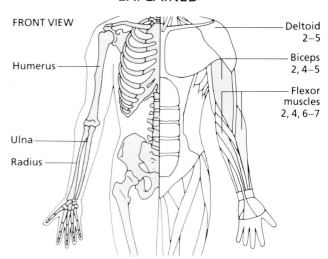

FRONT VIEW

Humerus

Ulna

Radius

Deltoid 2–5

Biceps 2, 4–5

Flexor muscles 2, 4, 6–7

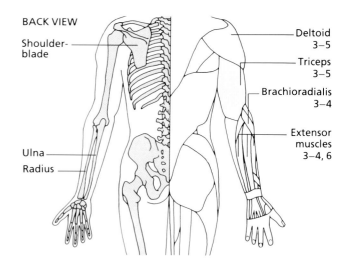

BACK VIEW

Shoulder-blade

Ulna

Radius

Deltoid 3–5

Triceps 3–5

Brachioradialis 3–4

Extensor muscles 3–4, 6

Numbers refer to steps in the following sequence, showing at which stage each muscle is worked upon.

The deltoid muscle gives the shoulder its rounded contour and moves the arm away from the body. It inserts into the shaft of the humerus, the upper-arm bone. At its lower end, the humerus forms the elbow joint, which is moved by two main muscles: the biceps at the front and the triceps behind. The flexor and extensor muscles of the forearm also rise from the humerus and work to move the wrist and the fingers. The brachioradialis muscle again stems from the humerus and inserts into the radius, which, like the ulna, is one of the forearm bones.

Arms

The opening movement (*see below*) is designed to encourage a person to open out. Your aim is to lift out the shoulder-blade to create more room and expansion in the upper body and shoulder area. With this in mind, the full-length effleurage includes gliding around the shoulder before pulling down the arm. The squeezing, kneading stroke on the upper arms (*see step 4, page 110*) is excellent for releasing tension or blocked emotions. My own experience here is of working with a client and beginning to feel quite angry myself. On asking her if she was angry at anything in her life, she revealed that she would really like to hit someone! She had summoned up aggression and anger, and held it in her upper arm instead of giving vent to it.

Your partner is lying down and covered up, except for the arm you are working on, throughout this sequence.

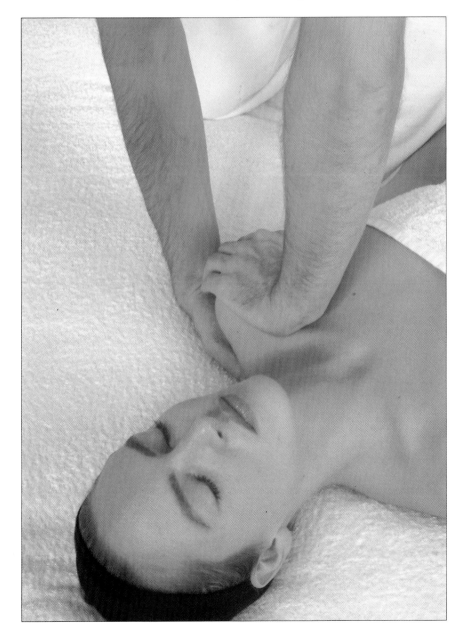

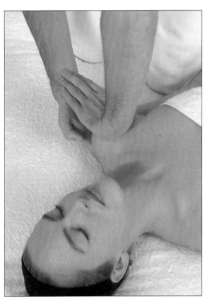

1 Use very little oil for this stroke. Kneel next to your partner's elbow, facing her head. Lift the shoulder with both hands to secure one hand beneath the shoulder-blade. Your fingers should be just touching the spine. If your partner raises her shoulder, press it down gently (*see left*). Place your hand flat on her upper chest, fingers pointing towards your arm. The heel of your hand should fit into the groove between chest and shoulder. Hold for 10 seconds. Breathe in, and as you breathe out, lean slightly into your upper hand as you squeeze both hands together to pull your hands slowly off the edge of the shoulder (*see above*). Repeat.

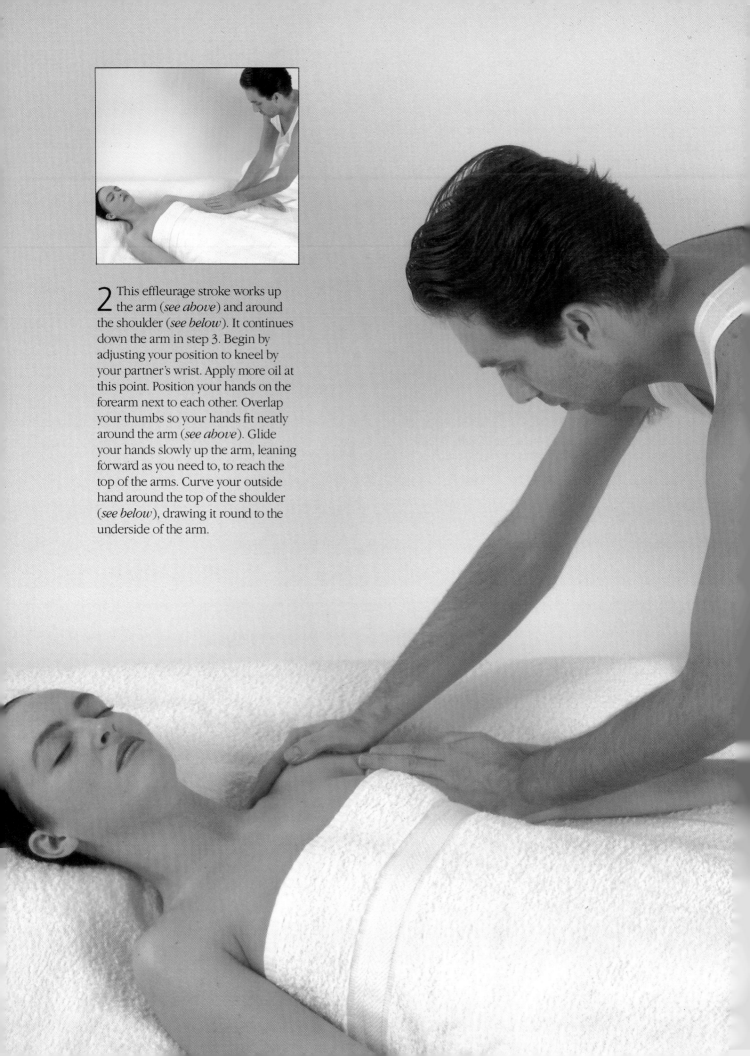

2 This effleurage stroke works up the arm (*see above*) and around the shoulder (*see below*). It continues down the arm in step 3. Begin by adjusting your position to kneel by your partner's wrist. Apply more oil at this point. Position your hands on the forearm next to each other. Overlap your thumbs so your hands fit neatly around the arm (*see above*). Glide your hands slowly up the arm, leaning forward as you need to, to reach the top of the arms. Curve your outside hand around the top of the shoulder (*see below*), drawing it round to the underside of the arm.

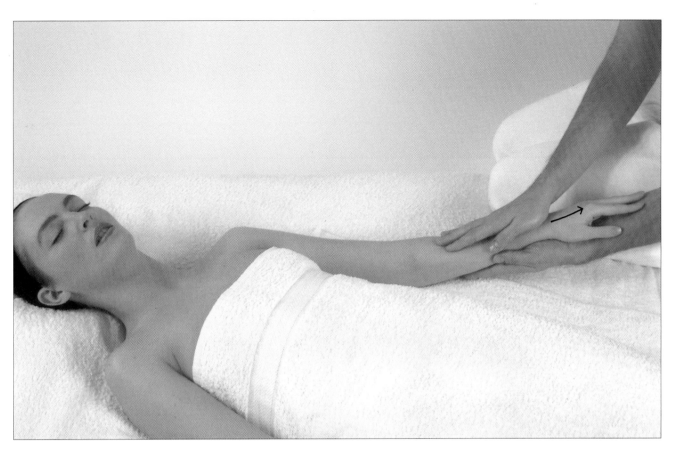

3 From the previous movement your hands are at the top of the arm – one on top, one underneath. Pull both hands slowly down the arm, over the hand and off (*see above*). Take care to place the hand gently on the floor as you take your hands off.

4 Cup your hands around the forearm, fingers pointing in opposite directions (*see left*). Glide your hands up the arm to the shoulder. Curve your upper hand around the shoulder and underneath the arm to draw both hands down the arm exactly as you did with the previous stroke.

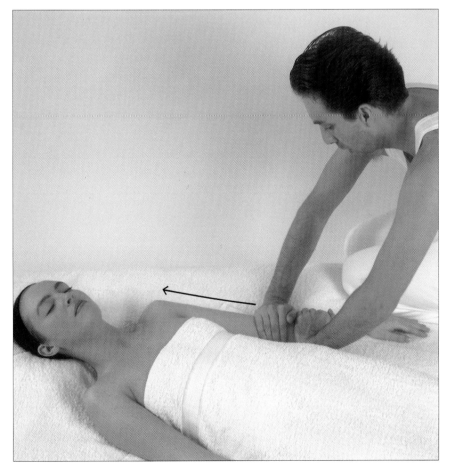

5 Hold your partner's arm on the inside of the elbow, letting her forearm rest on yours (*see right*). Lean your other hand into the outside of her upper arm to squeeze the flesh and muscle. Make sure that you lean in deeply to reach the muscles, otherwise you may simply be pinching the flesh. Work evenly over as much of the upper arm as you can reach, as far up as the shoulder and down to the elbow.

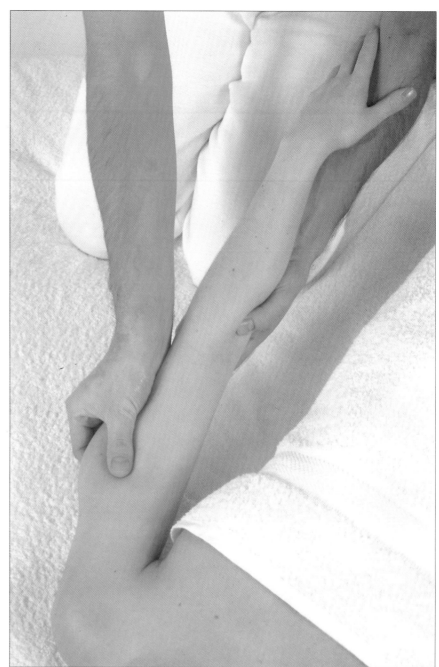

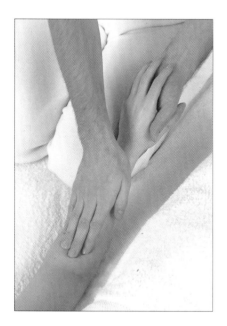

6 Hold your partner's hand in yours. Glide your other hand up the forearm to the elbow (*see above*). At the elbow, twist your hand around and glide your fingers down the underside of the forearm to the wrist. Apply firm and reassuring pressure, taking care not to push the arm down as you lean in. Hold the hand in a comfortable, supportive clasp, neither gripping it nor letting it flap. Repeat.

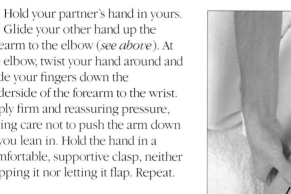

7 Continue holding the hand in the same position. Clasp your hand around the underside of the forearm, and place your thumb on top, facing sideways, just above the wrist. Breathe in, and as you breathe out, lean into your thumb and glide it up the arm to the elbow (*see left*). At the elbow, twist your hand around and glide down as you did with the previous stroke. Repeat. If you are completing the sequence here, 'ground' your partner by moving to the feet and holding them for at least 20 seconds.

Additional Sequence

If you are short of time but do not want to leave the arms out of a massage treatment, this sequence is ideal. It can take no longer than 5 minutes to do well and to make a noticeable difference. Alternatively, you can simply add it on to the previous routine to achieve a very thorough arms treatment. It is also a wonderfully beneficial sequence in its own right.

Its important contributions are to expand and open out the upper body, and to direct tension or blocked energy down the arms and through the hands. When you work on a specific part of the body it helps to have a purpose in mind to empower what you do. So, when carrying out the following routine, think of yourself as not only releasing tension in the arms themselves but attracting tension from the chest, throat and shoulder to be channelled out of the body through the arms.

These steps involve more active movement than any other sequence. It is vital that you hold the hands firmly and confidently without expecting your partner to do anything. This is especially true with step 3 (*see page 113*) when you lift the arms to stretch the shoulders. It is also extremely important to make sure that you have removed all oil from your hands; otherwise your hands will glide off.

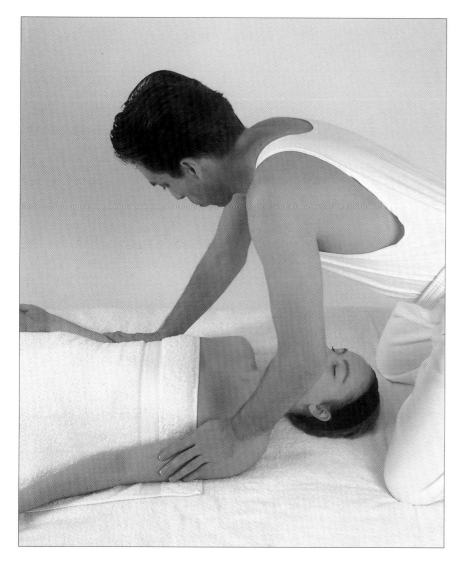

1 Kneel directly behind your partner's head. Place your hands on her upper arms, and lean in just enough to make a comfortable impact. Too much pressure will push the arms into the floor and feel painful. Clasp the arms firmly but avoid pinching. 'Walk' down the arms, lifting your hands slightly with each step. Continue down the arms until you reach the wrists. Walk back up the arms in exactly the same way, retracing your steps.

111

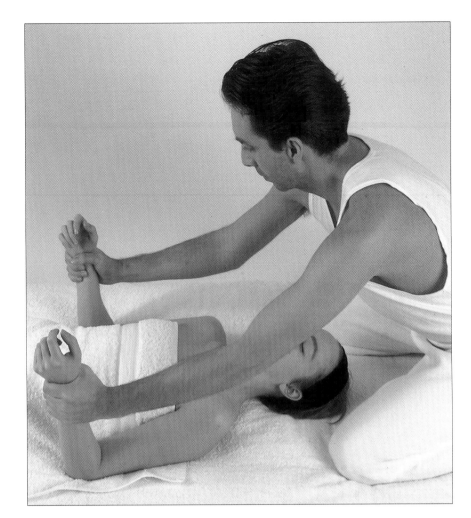

2 'Walk' down the arms again with your hands until you reach the wrists. Take hold of your partner's wrists (*see right*) and lift the arms up to bring them back to your lap. Hold your partner's hands in your hands (*see below*). Breathe in, and as you breathe out, lean back, gradually taking your partner's arms with you. Make sure that you check with your partner that the stretch is both comfortable and sufficient. If your partner needs more, accommodate this by moving your knees further back, releasing the arms and leaning back once again. Hold the stretch for at least 20 seconds.

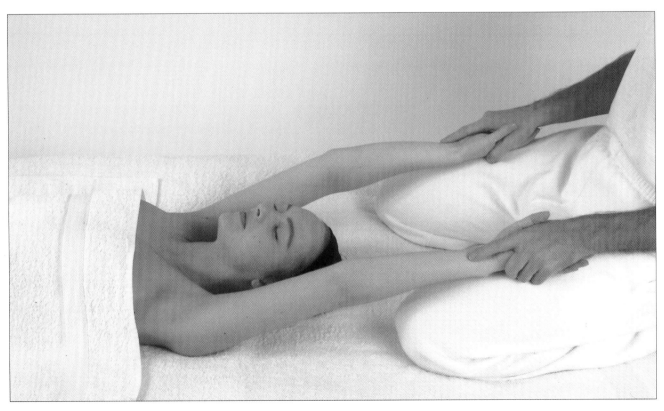

3 From the previous position, stand up, continuing to hold the hands with as little disturbance to your partner as possible. Stand directly behind her head. Breathe in, and as you breathe out, lean over to one side, taking your partner's arm with you, until her shoulder rises slightly off the floor (*see below*). Breathe in, and as you breathe out, lean to the other side taking your partner's arm with you again. Repeat this movement three times on each side.

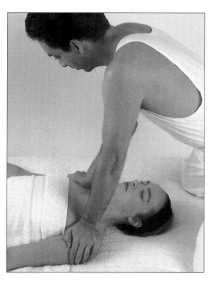

4 To complete the sequence, return to the kneeling position behind the head. Lean the heels of your hands into the hollow between the chest and shoulder, wrapping your fingers around the joint (*see above*). Breathe in, and as you breathe out, bring your body forward to lean on the heels of your hands. Graduate the pressure to encourage the chest area to widen, and the shoulders to lower to the floor without discomfort. Remember to end by 'grounding' your partner, moving to the feet and holding them for at least 20 seconds.

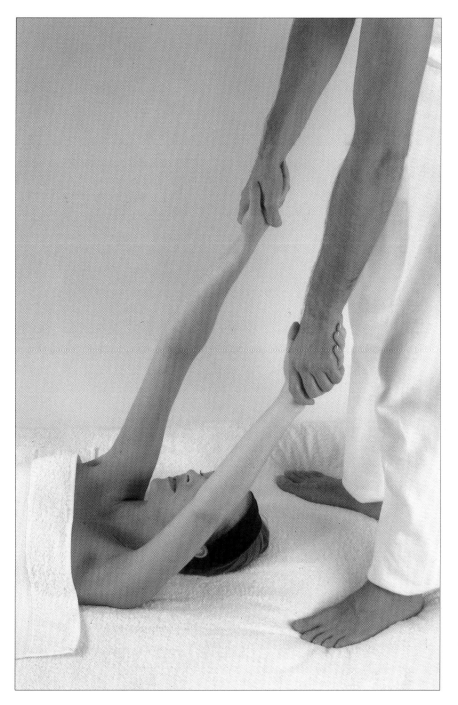

Hands

You can massage a hand just about anywhere, any time – on a long journey, watching a film, visiting a friend in hospital – the list is endless. You can also work directly on the skin without your partner having to take any clothes off. This may be an important consideration for someone who is nervous of receiving massage, or is rarely touched. When I was training in massage, I gained immense experience at the hands of my friends!

The sequence is also highly suitable to give to elderly friends and neighbours. Such people may be living alone and receiving no physical contact whatsoever, so massage can be hugely benefi-cial. We could all make a huge difference to the quality of life for the elderly if we were to visit neighbours or the elderly in hospital to carry out this simple routine. Try it and see.

If you are working on the hands as a continua-tion of the arms sequence, include it before the additional arms routine. You need very little oil and your partner may prefer you to use a favourite hand lotion instead. The skin on the hands is the thinnest and shows signs of age before anywhere else on the body. Working in a luxurious oil or cream and increasing circulation to the area will contribute to keeping hands healthy and youthful.

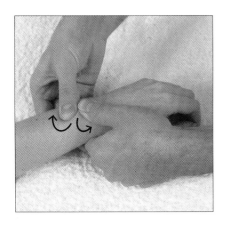

1 Hold your partner's hand in your hands to leave your thumbs free to work on her wrist (*see above*). Use the ball of your thumbs to lean into the bony area of the wrist, and slowly rotate in between and over the bones. Work slowly and precisely in this way, all along the wrist.

2 Wrap your hands around your partner's hand, bringing the heels of your hands onto the back of her hand (*see right*). Breathe in, and as you breathe out, lean into your heels as they glide firmly across the hand in opposite directions. Return your hands to their original position and repeat. If you wish, you can add variety to this stroke by using only one hand at a time.

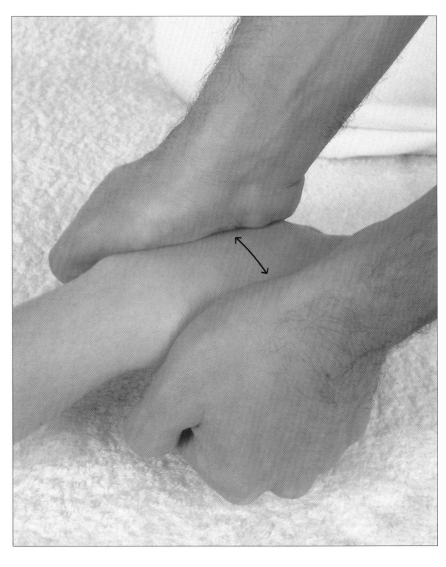

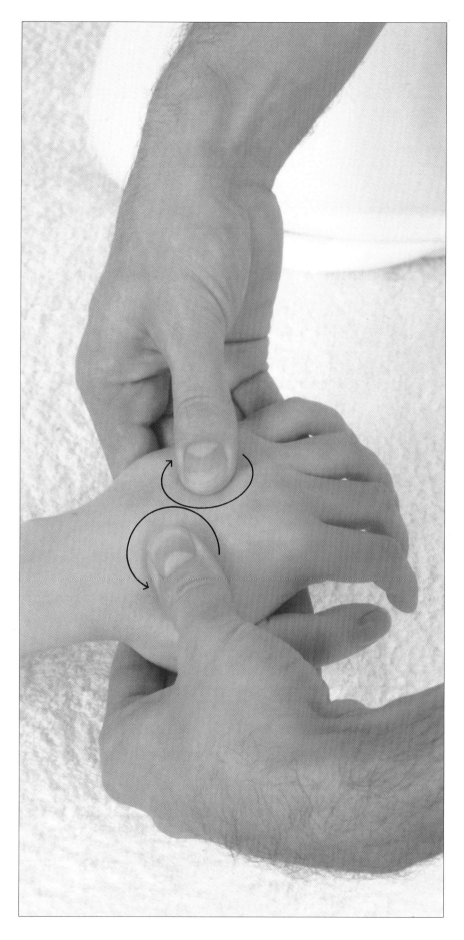

3 Do not use this stroke on pregnant women as this area houses a powerful acupressure point for elimination. Wrap your fingers around your partner's palms leaving your thumbs free to work on the back of the hand (*see left*). Hold the hand firmly or rest it on your lap. Lean into and slowly rotate your thumbs in small circles over the back of the hand. Lift them off slightly at the end of each circle to move on to cover the rest of the back of the hand. Finally, come to the web between the thumb and forefinger (*see below*). Lean your thumb into and circle this small area.

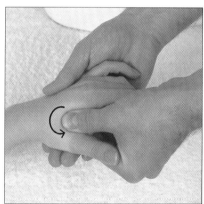

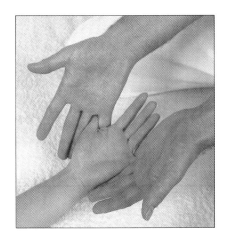

4 Insert your partner's thumb between your little finger and ring finger. Insert her little finger between the little finger and ring finger of your other hand (*see above*). Stretch the palms as you do this. Tuck your fingers under the back of her hand. Lean your thumbs in and rotate in small circles over the palm (*see right*).

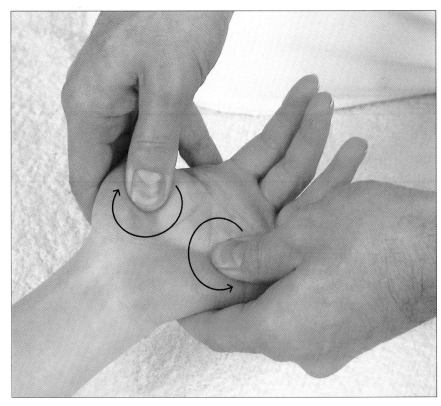

5 Hold your partner's hand in yours (*see right*). Lean your thumb into the valley between the bones on the back of the hand leading up from the fingers to the wrist. Glide up each valley to the wrist. Begin in the valley from the little finger, and move on to work up each of the valleys until you have covered all four of them.

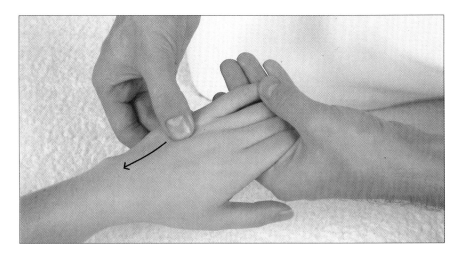

6 Clasp your partner's hand in yours (*see right*). Take hold of the little finger, right down at the base, between your thumb and forefinger. Squeeze it as your fingers slide firmly up to the tip. Here, squeeze and pinch the finger as you pull your fingers off. Work along each finger in turn, ending on the thumb.

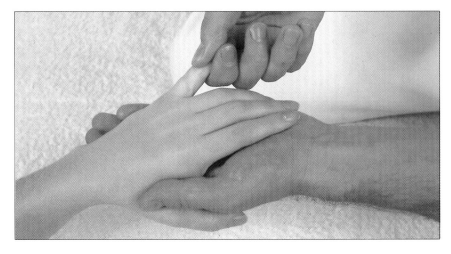

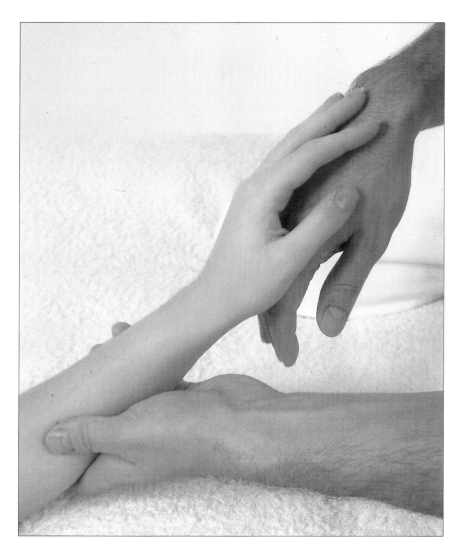

7 To complete this sequence, hold your partner's forearm with one hand. Slide the back of your other hand under her forearm to glide up under her hand (*see left*). Pull your hand up to insert your fingers firmly between hers (*see below*). While clasping the fingers firmly with yours, pull your fingers up and back towards you. Repeat twice. This is a wonderful stroke, which your partner will love. Do persevere if you find it difficult initially. You only need to get it right once and you will have mastered it forever. If you are completing your treatment here, remember to 'ground' your partner by holding the feet for at least 20 seconds.

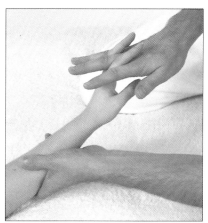

Common Ailments

Before you massage your partner, always ask if there are any physical problems. The following is a list of the most common complaints of the arms and hands you are likely to come across. These are likely to be caused by a specific problem, rather than general tension.

● **Fractures**
A fractured wrist and forearm can benefit from massage, but make sure that you treat it only after recovery. Work deeply to break up any scar tissue, to relieve pain and to mobilize the joint. Using lavender, marjoram and rosemary essential oils will help to soothe aching and promote healing.

● **Lymphodema**
This occurs as a result of a mastectomy where the auxiliary lymph nodes are removed. The result is serious swelling in the arms with a backlog of lymph fluid trapped there, since it can no longer be processed by the lymph nodes in the armpit. Massage is extremely useful here to help pump the fluid out of the arm. Use firm effleurage strokes to get the fluid moving. Hold the arm up to encourage this, or raise it on some pillows so you can work with both hands. Oils renowned for clearing the lymphatic system include geranium, lavender and juniper.

● **Tennis Elbow**
This is caused by overuse and manifests as an inflammation on the outside of the elbow. The best remedy is rest when it is most painful. The most we can do is to help to maintain mobility in the elbow joint. Carry out the entire sequence but work with your thumbs around the elbow itself rotating and pressing in as deeply as your partner can tolerate. Anti-inflammatory and pain relieving oils such as camomile, rosemary and lavender can also help. Golfer's Elbow is the same except that it occurs on the inside of the elbow.

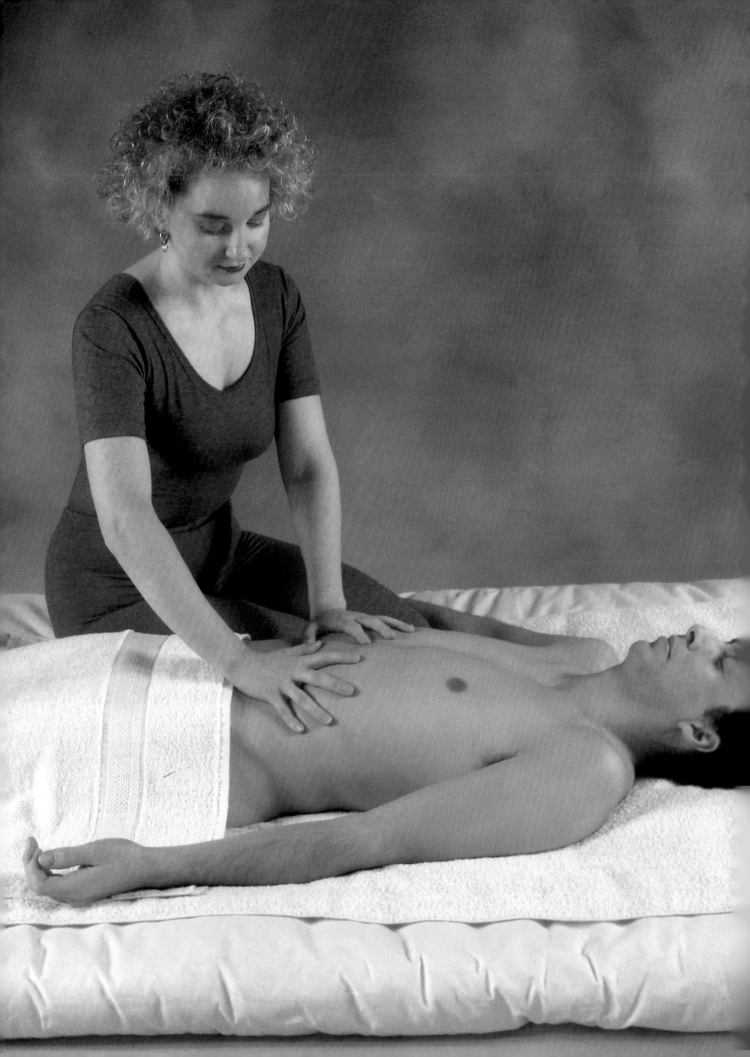

7

Abdomen

The abdomen is the most vulnerable and unprotected area of the body. Within this tender cavity sit the vital organs, not least our intestines or 'guts'. It is here that our raw emotions and passions originate, before spreading out through the rest of our body to find expression. We speak of our 'gut feeling' as our true feeling, our instinct. We trust it to bypass the logic of our minds, to reveal the truth. When we are shaken to our core, terrified or angry, we involuntarily empty our stomachs. Our insides feel 'tied up in knots' when we are worried and anxious, making it difficult to eat. We cut ourselves off from this vital centre by breathing only from the upper chest, blocking off access to any uncomfortable feelings, and depriving ourselves of the extra life energy deeper breathing would bring.

Oriental medical philosophy understands that the abdomen is far more than an area of the body. They speak of the 'hara' as the house of our vital energy, the seat of consciousness (in place of the mind). In Japan, *ampaku* is a specific massage practised on the hara or abdomen to diagnose and treat serious illnesses. Skilled practitioners with many years experience can work directly on the energy of the vital organs and processes of the body in this way.

When abdominal massage is done well and with care, it is the most comforting and relaxing experience imaginable. Be reassuring and confident in your touch to bring your partner awareness of his or her instinctive consciousness.

The abdomen houses powerful
feelings such as anger, rage and jealousy.
Soothing, caring massage here can help us
to integrate such feelings and to spread
waves of relaxation throughout
our entire mind and body.

Abdomen

The abdomen is the area at the front of the body from the pelvis up to the ribs. It is separated from the thoracic cavity, which contains the lungs and heart, by a sheet of muscle known as the diaphragm. This muscle is an important component of respiration, contracting on inspiration and pulling its central portion downwards, thus increasing the capacity of the thoracic cavity. At the same time, the abdominal contents become somewhat compressed. These include the stomach and spleen, liver and gall-bladder, pancreas, large and small intestines and the bladder.

The abdominal muscles form a strong, supportive covering whose functions include flexing and rotating the trunk, maintaining normal pelvic tilt and controlling intra-abdominal pressure, which is an important factor in supporting the spine. These activities are critical to good and efficient use of the spine and to producing balanced movement of the whole body. If there is weakness in the abdominal region, it will lead to instability of the lumbar spine and, furthermore, to a tendency to place excessive strain onto the lumbar muscles.

The digestive system is essentially a simple tube, linking the mouth to the rectum. There are specialized areas at various sections of the tract to help the digestion of specific types of food. The walls of the intestines are highly muscular, the contraction of which produces the movement of the food through the tract while it is acted on by the digestive processes. This is known as peristalsis. Proper functioning of the digestive system is assisted by movement and activity in the body, and massage can be of great benefit in helping to stimulate a sluggish system. If the intestinal muscles are tense, peristalsis and elimination will be impeded, resulting in constipation and possibly abdominal bloating. Previous surgery could also lead to the formation of adhesions and fibrous scar tissue. These can cause pain and can also inhibit the efficiency of digestion.

THE ABDOMEN MUSCLES EXPLAINED

FRONT VIEW

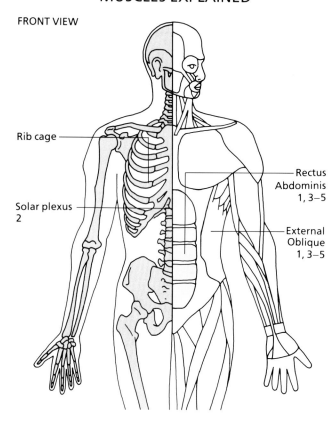

Rib cage

Solar plexus 2

Rectus Abdominis 1, 3–5

External Oblique 1, 3–5

Numbers refer to steps in the following sequence, showing at which stage each muscle is worked upon.

It is possible to show only a few of the abdominal muscles and their relationships to each other here as many of them are situated quite deeply. The organs housed in the abdomen are supported by three layers of superficial muscles. The deepest layer of muscle in the abdomen is called the Transversus Abdominis. It runs horizontally across the abdomen, with a corset-like effect. Superficial to this lie the internal and external oblique muscles. Their fibres pass diagonally across the body to insert into a central sheet of fascia: several layers of muscle fibres and sheets of fibrous tissue at the back of the abdomen. The most superficial of these muscles is the Rectus Abdominis, the corrugations of which may be seen in people with athletic build. Its muscle fibres extend vertically, from the lower ribs to the rim of the pelvis. The solar plexus is an area at the pit of the stomach where large numbers of nerve fibres meet.

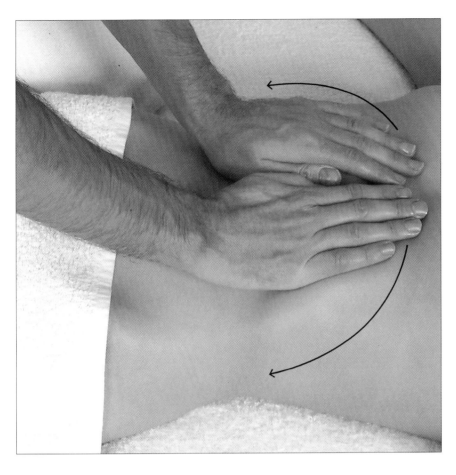

1 Kneel alongside your partner's torso, so that your leg makes contact, but do not lean into your partner. Bring your hands gently down to make contact on the abdomen. Keep your hands quite light, allowing your partner's abdomen to rise and fall with each breath. Hold here for 20 seconds, then bring your hands off gradually to apply the oil. Gently return your hands to rest above the navel (*see top left*). Glide your hands around slowly to either side of the torso. Pull them up onto the lower abdomen (*see bottom left*) and push up the centre back to your original starting position, in one smooth movement (*see below*). Repeat five times. Keep the pressure quite light and, above all, keep the movement very slow. Allow your own hands to stay relaxed throughout and breathe comfortably yourself.

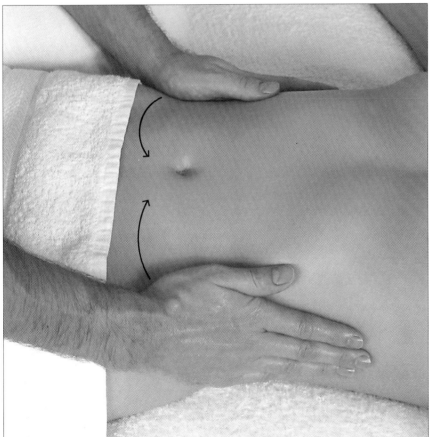

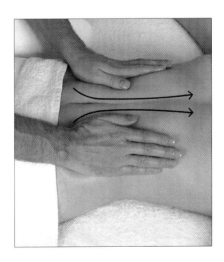

121

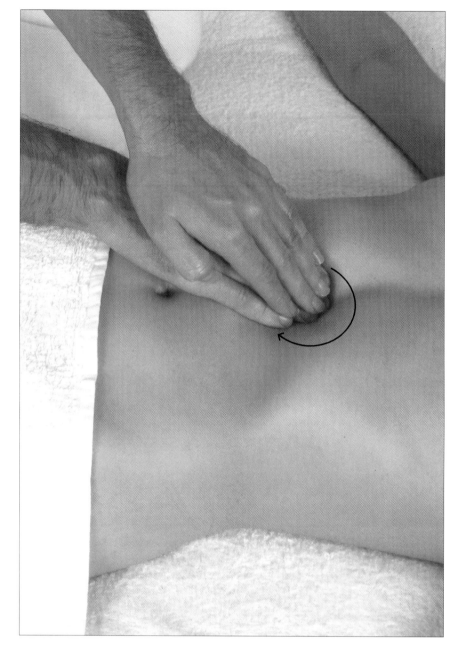

2 Place one hand on top of the other. Relax your hands and place the length of your fingers down flat on the solar plexus: the triangle formed by the sides of the rib cage. Glide your hands smoothly around this area in a slow, circular motion (*see right*). Repeat five times. This is a collecting area for tension and worry. If the large diaphragm muscle, which lies around and under the rib-cage, contracts and shortens through tension, it intensifies the shallow breathing cycle. Slow, reassuring effleurage can help to release the diaphragm and deepen the breathing.

3 Place one hand on top of the other, and glide them down flat, so that your whole hand is in contact. Begin on the side of the abdomen nearest you. Breathe in, and as you breathe out, lean slightly into your hands as you push them up the side of the abdomen (*see left*). Continue to push around the centre of the abdomen and down the far side. At the bottom, curve your hands around so the heels of your hands face you as you pull back towards you (*see right*). Repeat five times. Work very slowly and deeper than you did with the previous effleurage.

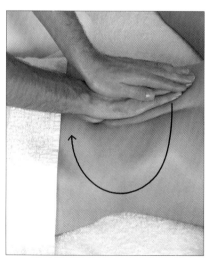

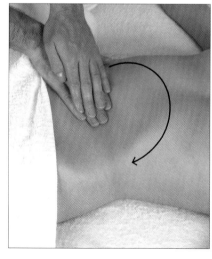

4 Move around to kneel facing your partner's abdomen. Place one hand on the side of the abdomen nearest to you and the other across on the other side, hooked over the side of the torso. Breathe in, and as you breathe out, push the hand nearest you away towards the far side. At the same time, pull your other hand back towards you. This movement needs to be slow, strong and thorough. Use your body-weight to bring impact to your hands, as you draw them rhythmically across and over the sides of the abdomen (*see below*). Cover the entire length of the abdomen.

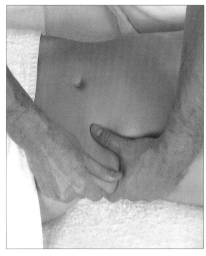

5 Begin by kneading on the edge of the abdomen furthest away from you, coming up on your knees to lean into your hands. Place both hands down, fingers facing each other. Lean one hand in to scoop up flesh between your fingers and thumb (*see above*). Push this hand towards the other and immediately begin the same movement with that hand. Set up a flowing rhythm and keep the movement slow and thorough. As you complete the side furthest away from you, move onto the centre of the abdomen and finally lean back to work on the side nearest you (*see below*). The slow kneading motion should feel pleasant and relaxing to your partner. To reassure yourself, it might be a good idea to check quietly with your partner that the depth and speed of the movement feel comfortable.

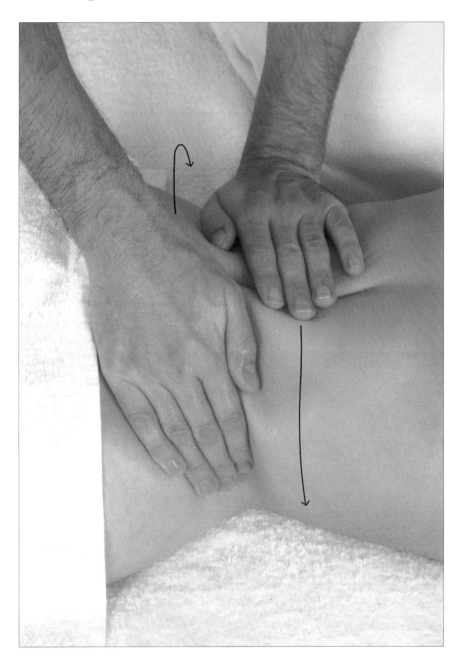

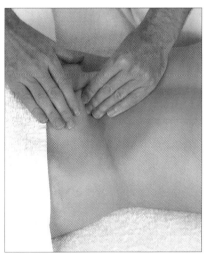

Additional Sequence

The following sequence is an excellent way to deepen your partner's breathing. In times of acute anxiety, as we breathe less deeply, we use our lungs less and the muscles around them (especially the diaphragm) shrink, making further relaxed breathing even more difficult. This contributes to a syndrome of chronic, low-level anxiety, reducing our potential to experience and enjoy life fully. Releasing tension from the diaphragm is, therefore, a valuable way of restoring a sense of balance and harmony to the whole person, physically and emotionally.

The whole-torso effleurage in this section soothes the abdomen and connects it with the upper torso. As you work, you can encourage your partner to breathe with the flow and movement of your hands. When you bring your hands to the abdomen, pause, then quietly ask your partner to breathe in. As you feel the abdomen rise, move your hands slowly up to the chest.

Here, ask her to breathe out and as she does, sweep your hands down the sides of the torso or the arms. Continue to give directions for three more movements and by then your partner will be following the movement of your hands automatically. When I do this stroke, I like to think of moving any tension on unresolved emotions up and out of the body, especially when I work down the arms and off at the hands.

This sequence can be added easily to the end of the previous one. You simply adjust your position to kneel alongside your partner's abdomen. If your partner is female, what you need to consider is whether she would be happy to expose her body for this stroke. If you are male, you also need to check whether you feel comfortable with this level of contact.

This routine is invaluable if you have concentrated on the back of the body but wanted to make contact with the front.

1 Kneel alongside your partner's abdomen. Apply oil to your hands. Place your hands gently on the sides of the abdomen. Breathe in, and as you breathe out, lean into your hands with your body-weight and slowly glide them across to the centre of the abdomen. Here, push your hands up towards the chest. On women, before you reach the breasts, discreetly place one hand on top of the other to push up through the centre. If you have completed the previous sequence your pressure here can be quite strong and dynamic. Make sure, however, that your hands are relaxed and that all the movements are very slow. Remind yourself to breathe, to stay relaxed and, if you are unsure about your pressure, check quietly with your partner.

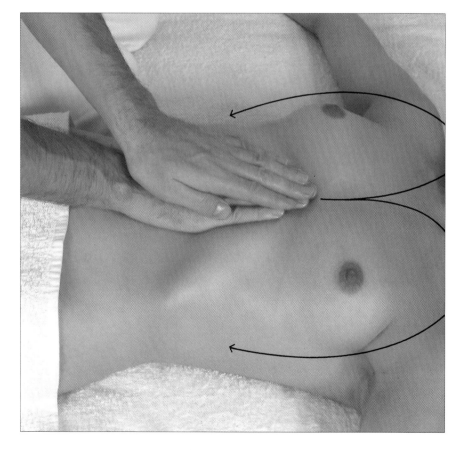

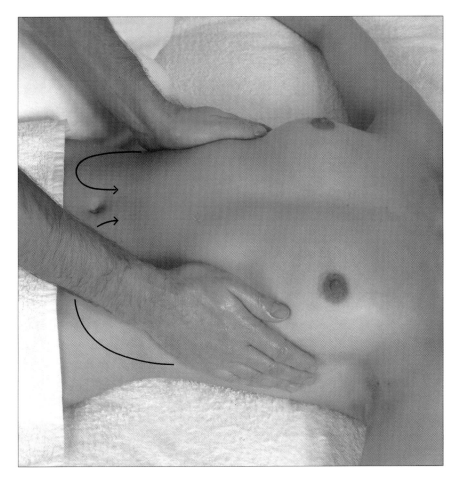

2 From the first part of this stroke, your hands will be on the chest, one hand on top of the other. Separate the hands and pull them across the chest towards the arms. At the arms, pull your hands down onto the sides of the torso. Pull around to the centre of the abdomen and repeat the stroke from the beginning of step 1. Repeat the full stroke three times. As a variation here, instead of pulling your hands down the sides of the torso, you can bring them onto the upper arms and pull down the length of the arms. Be careful to re-establish contact on the abdomen gently and sensitively.

Common Ailments

Before you start to massage your partner, always ask if there are any physical problems. The following is a list of the most common abdominal complaints you are likely to come across. It tells you what the best course of action is in each case: whether or not a massage would help and when medical attention is advisable.

● **Abdominal Bloating**
This usually indicates water retention, a food allergy or faulty digestion and elimination. Your partner needs to consult both a homoeopath and a dietary therapist. Concentrate on effleurage strokes, moving deeply in the direction of the colon, and use marjoram or rosemary oils. If the problem is water retention specifically, then concentrate on the

kneading strokes to help move the fluid out of the tissues. Use juniper, geranium or rosemary oil here.

● **Constipation**
Massage is a very pleasant and effective means of relieving the bloatedness, abdominal pains and headaches that accompany constipation. The whole sequence is useful but emphasize steps 2 and 3 (see page 122) and use juniper, rosemary and marjoram oils. If it is chronic, your partner should consult a dietary therapist.

● **Hiatus Hernia**
This condition is stress-related and occurs when part of the stomach pushes up into the thoracic cavity, causing pain and damage to the lining of the oesophagus. Make sure your partner's head is propped up, to encourage the juices to flow

downwards, and use peppermint, lavender, camomile or neroli oil.

● **Indigestion**
Nervous tension, anxiety, eating rich foods, over-eating and over-drinking can all cause a stomach upset. Gentle, soothing massage especially with peppermint oil will help. Do all the strokes very slowly, leaving out the kneading and wringing. If the problem is persistent, your partner should consult an expert.

● **Menstrual Cramps**
Soothing, calming massage on the abdomen with camomile, lavender, rose and neroli oils is very effective. Work slowly, and as deeply as your partner can tolerate. You could suggest to your partner that she considers seeing an acupuncturist or homoeopath.

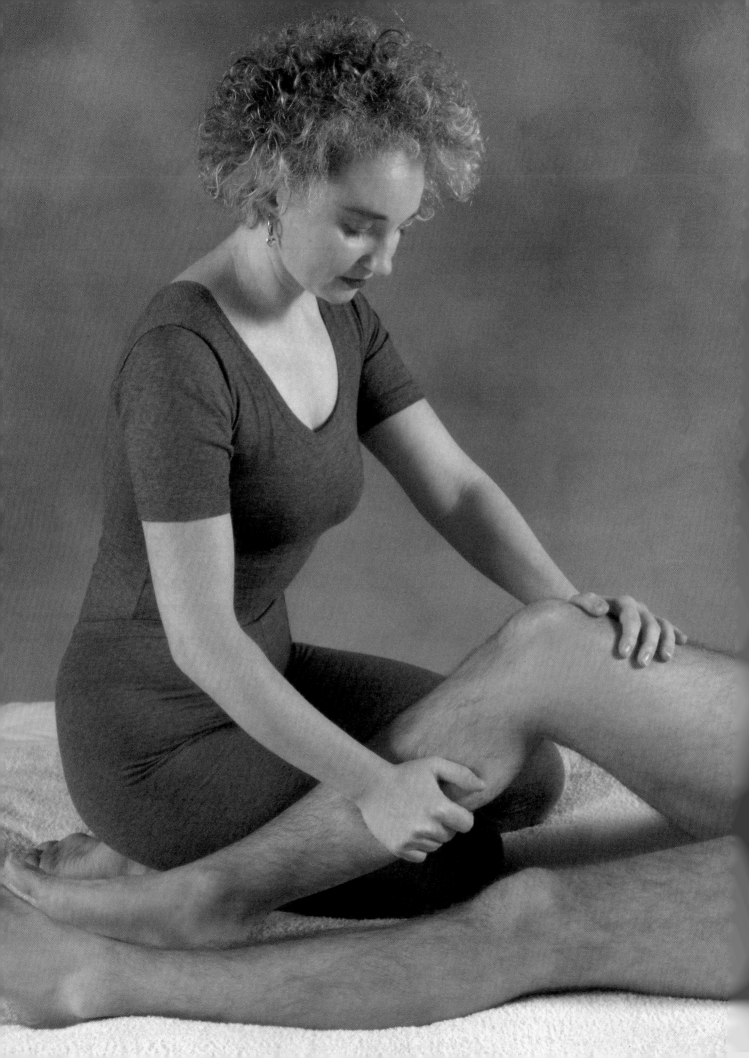

8

Front of Legs and Feet

Almost everyone appreciates and benefits from a front-of-legs routine. But for those who 'live in their heads' or with their 'head in the clouds', it is especially pertinent. Such individuals have a limited perspective – neither informed nor balanced – as their feet are not firmly on the ground. A good, thorough massage on the legs and feet helps to lessen such a mind–body split.

The way we hold our legs also reveals our feelings of safety within our world. A rigid stance with locked knees declares 'I will stand firm, I won't give in', or conversely 'I must hold myself together'. Such an outlook and accompanying physical response tends to become rigid and fixed. Physically, this results in loss of vitality in the legs and shortened, contracted, tense muscles.

Another association with the knee is fear. We speak of 'going weak at the knees' and our knees begin to shake when we are frightened. This experience corresponds with the traditional Chinese medicine system that links the knees to the kidneys where fear is the influential emotion.

Finally, working on the feet is doubly beneficial since you are, in effect, treating the entire body. The feet are covered with reflex areas which correspond to the organs and nerves of the body, and as you work you will automatically affect a much wider area than the feet alone.

*A good leg and foot massage encourages
a clearer perspective and a fresh outlook on
life. We feel more balanced, more connected
to the whole of our body and less
bound up in our head.*

Front of Legs and Feet

Massaging the front of legs and the feet brings great benefits to everyone. Athletes are particularly likely to find a massage treatment in this area a wonderful experience. The muscles of the front of legs and feet work extremely hard. We use them nearly all the time, to walk, run, crouch, sit down and stand up. Yet many of us misuse these essential muscles, storing tension in the lower-leg area. This prevents force from being evenly distributed along the leg and can cause painful conditions, such as shin splints. Massaging the calf muscles can break up this tension, and bring feelings of deep relaxation to the recipient.

The fleshy area of the inner thigh is made up of the adductor muscles and the large muscle groups of the quadriceps. The adductor muscles connect the front of the pelvis to the femur. They are responsible for drawing the legs together. We use these muscles, for example, to carry out a breat-stroke kick while swimming. More importantly, they stabilize the trunk and control the rotation of the femur during walking. Tightness in these muscles causes an alteration in gait which may lead to hip, knee or sacro-iliac problems.

The quadriceps is composed of four distinct muscles, three of which are attached to the shaft of the femur. The other one rises from the pelvis. The muscles combine at their lower end to form the patella tendon within which lies the patellar or kneecap. The tendon finally inserts into the upper part of the tibia. This muscle controls knee extension and is used in activities such as rising from a squatting position.

The feet are the base upon which our entire body rests. They connect us with the earth, bringing a sense of groundedness and balance. Massaging the feet is hugely beneficial. It helps to tone the muscles that perform the arduous task of supporting our entire body-weight and can also aid circulation in the feet.

The muscles that work on the foot and ankle are the anterior tibial muscles. Long tendons connect them to the bones of the feet. These

THE FRONT OF LEGS MUSCLES EXPLAINED

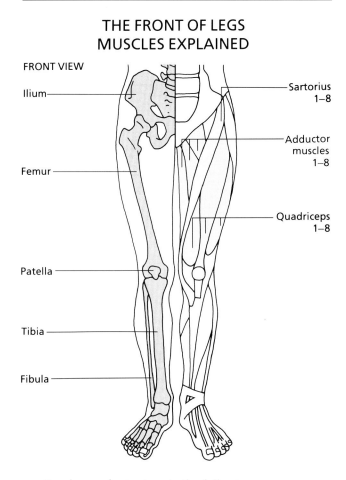

FRONT VIEW

Ilium

Femur

Patella

Tibia

Fibula

Sartorius 1–8

Adductor muscles 1–8

Quadriceps 1–8

Numbers refer to steps in the following sequence, showing at which stage each muscle is worked upon.

The long bones of the leg – the femur, tibia and fibula – are crossed by large and powerful muscles. The upper end of the femur forms the hip joint with the hip bone, the ilium part of which can be felt by placing a hand on the hip. The fibula is a slender bone at the side of the tibia, which forms the lateral side of the ankle joint at its lower end. The quadriceps and the sartorius muscles lie on the front of the thigh and control extension of the patella (kneecap). The adductor muscles are found in the inner-thigh area and work to stabilize the body during walking.

muscles move the unsupported foot. Working in reverse, they control the position of the body on the weight-bearing foot. They also help to maintain the arches of the foot to give it its important shock-absorbing quality.

Front of Legs

The front-of-legs sequence includes some of the strokes you used on the back of the legs. The obvious difference is that you have to work around the knee, the shin-bone and the ankle-bone, avoiding direct pressure on the shin-bone and the knee.

Most people thoroughly enjoy the strokes on the knees (*see steps 9 and 10, page 133*), although occasionally you may work on a partner who finds them uncomfortable. If so, be aware of your partner's reaction and use light effleurage around the knee instead.

As with the back of the legs, the thighs benefit from firm, slow, deep strokes. To ensure deep enough pressure, place your body correctly so you can lean into the stroke, particularly when kneading (*see step 4, page 130*) and applying petrissage (*see step 5, page 131*).

Your position is kneeling throughout the sequence, so you may want to support yourself with a pillow between the back of your thighs and your calves. Your partner may appreciate a pillow under her knees to take pressure off the pelvis. I recommend that you cover the leg you are not working on, to ensure that your partner does not feel cold or too exposed. Remember also to avoid working too far up into the inner thigh with any of the strokes.

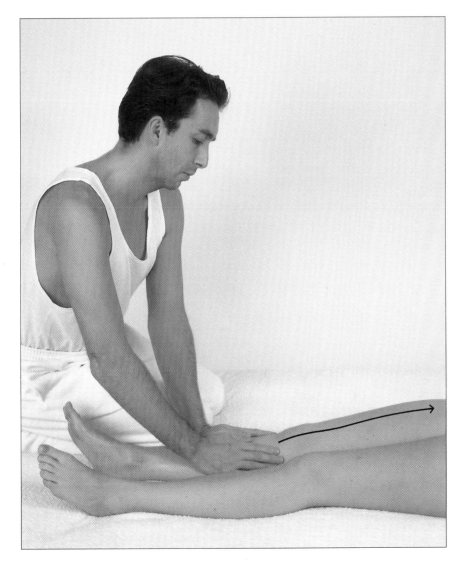

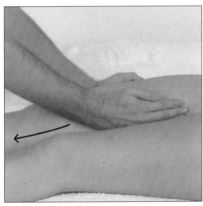

1 Kneel alongside your partner's ankles. Apply the oil to your hands and make contact with the lower leg (*see left*). Breathe in, and as you breathe out, lean into your hands, pushing them up the leg. Glide very lightly, with no pressure at all, over the knee. As you approach the thigh, you may need to lean up on your knees to reach the entire length of the thigh, and to give you more body-weight to drop into your stroke. When you reach the top of the thigh, curve your outside hand around the outside of the leg. Take your inside hand only as far up the leg as you feel is comfortable for your partner. Draw both hands down the sides of the leg to complete this smooth rhythmic movement (*see above*).

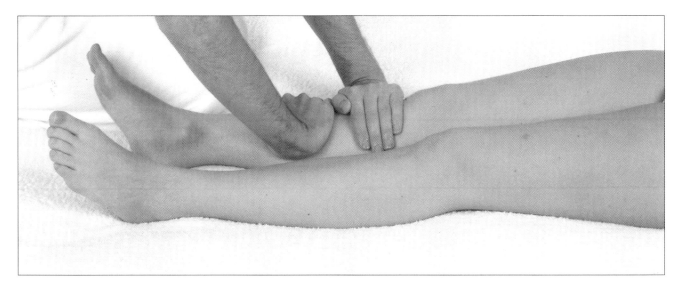

2 Cup your hands around the lower
leg, fingers pointing in opposite
directions (*see above*). Lean slightly
into your hands to avoid pressing
down on the shin-bone. Glide over
the knee. Lean up on your knees and
lean into the thigh. Curve your hands
around the upper leg and draw them
down the sides to the ankle.

3 Place your hands on the thigh just
above the knee. Lean your weight
into the thigh (*see right*). To finish,
draw your hands back to the knee.

4 Change your position to kneel,
facing your partner's thigh (*see
below*). Place your hands side by side.
Lean into one hand, pick up and
squeeze the flesh and muscle
between fingers and thumb. Push
towards your other hand as it begins
the same movement. Continue slowly
and rhythmically.

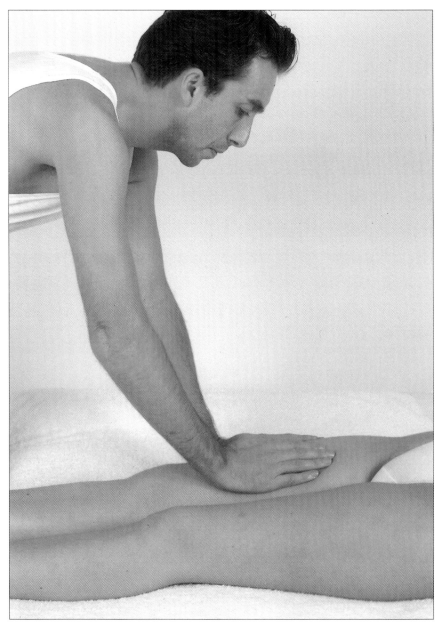

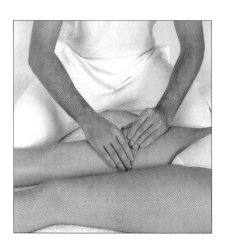

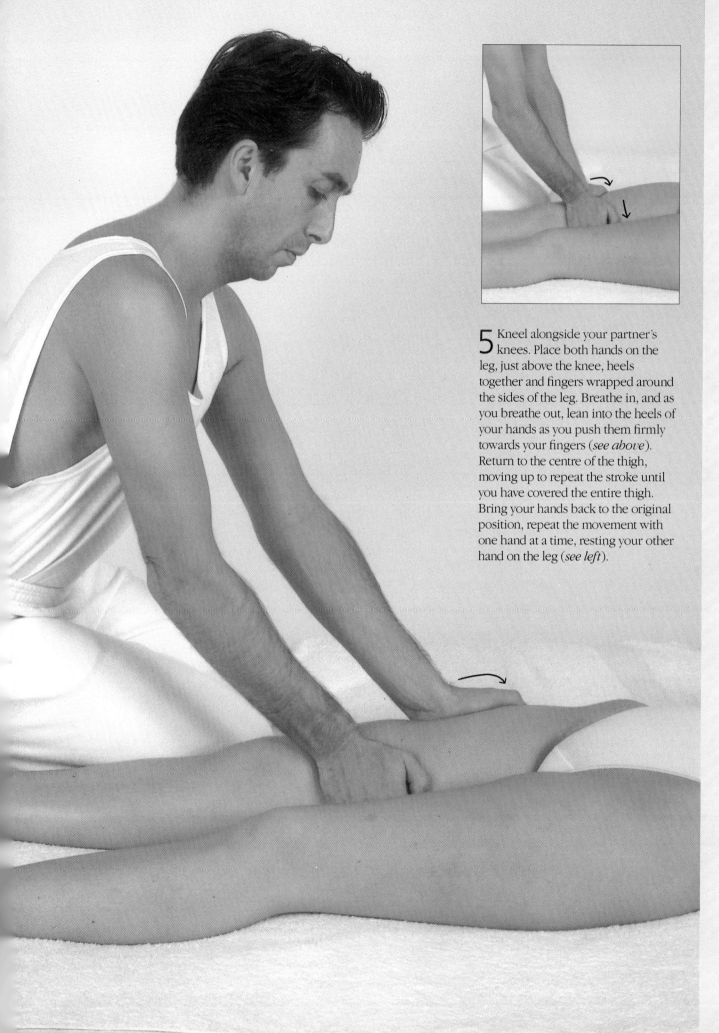

5 Kneel alongside your partner's knees. Place both hands on the leg, just above the knee, heels together and fingers wrapped around the sides of the leg. Breathe in, and as you breathe out, lean into the heels of your hands as you push them firmly towards your fingers (*see above*). Return to the centre of the thigh, moving up to repeat the stroke until you have covered the entire thigh. Bring your hands back to the original position, repeat the movement with one hand at a time, resting your other hand on the leg (*see left*).

6 Kneel facing your partner's thigh. Place both hands down flat on the thigh, fingers pointing away from you. Breathe in, and as you breathe out, lean in and push one hand slowly and firmly across the thigh. Immediately begin to pull your other hand slowly back towards you (*see right*). Use your body-weight to bring impact to your hands and make sure that you are lifting up flesh and muscle as the hands criss-cross against each other, not simply sliding the hands over the skin. It needs to be a dynamic, deep and thorough movement. Continue this action until you have covered the entire thigh.

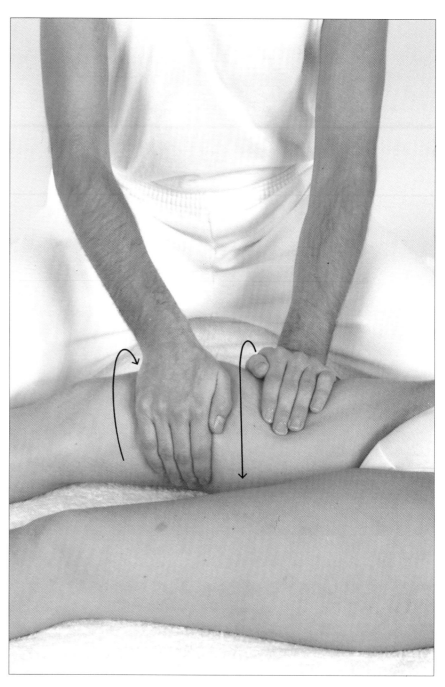

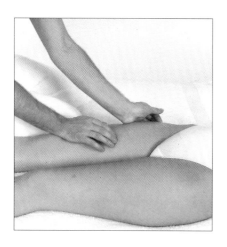

7 Change position to kneel alongside your partner's knees again. Place both hands flat on the leg just above the knee. Breathe in, and as you breathe out, lean into the heels of your hands. Push them one after the other up the centre of the thigh to the top (*see above*). Keep your fingers soft, relaxed and in contact with the leg. Repeat the movement on the outer thigh and the inner, beginning each time from the knee upwards. Keep the momentum slow, deep and thorough.

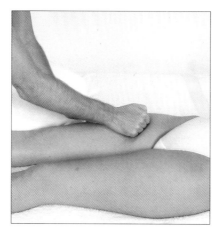

8 Make your hands into loose fists and place them on the leg just above the knee. Lean in slightly and push your knuckles, one after the other, up the leg to the top of the thigh (*see left*). Return your hands to their starting position and repeat the movement up the inner thigh and then, more gently, up the outer thigh. Remember that the outer thigh can be a very painful area so try to increase the pressure very gradually, and be particularly sensitive to your partner's response.

9 Wrap your hands under the knee, leaving your thumbs available to work around the joint. Begin at the top of the knee, leaning your thumbs gradually into the grooves around the outside of the knee pad itself (*see below*). Work out from the top of the knee around the sides, thumbs on either side, following the joint round to the bottom. Apply the pressure slowly, and only to a depth that feels comfortable to your partner. Focus the pressure inwards towards the centre of the knee, and maintain constant pressure for 5 seconds at each indentation.

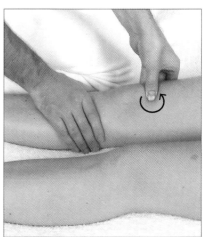

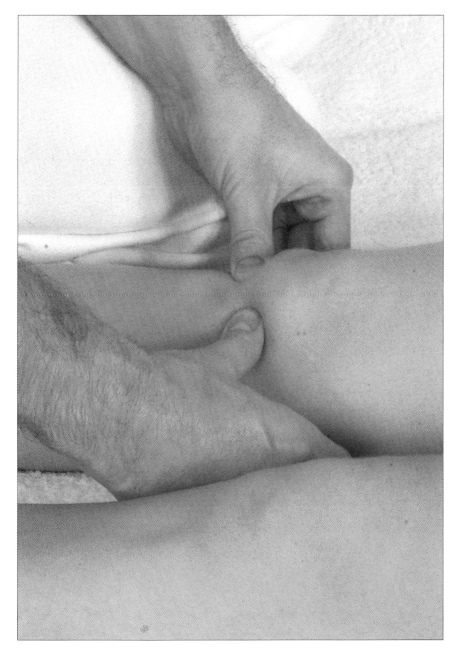

10 Rest one hand above the knee. Place your other hand on the knee with your thumb available to work on the knee. Lean into the spaces around the knee, slowly rotating your thumb (*see above*). You are working into the same grooves and indentations as the previous stroke, but rotating your thumb in slow circles instead of pressing in. If you are completing your treatment here, 'ground' your partner by moving to the feet and holding them for at least 20 seconds.

Feet

This routine for the feet is a natural addition to the front-of-legs sequence, and makes for a very thorough treatment. You will be working in a very small area, so you may not need to add any more oil to your hands. It is often a good idea to prop up your partner's foot on a pillow, to enable you to reach the sole of the foot without straining.

This sequence is also versatile enough to give independently of the leg sequence. For an exclusive foot massage, allow your partner to relax in a comfortable seat while you sit facing her, working on one foot at a time on your lap. It makes a wonderful treat to let the feet soak in a bowl of warm, scented water for a few minutes before the treatment. You will need, then, to dry the feet gently on a soft towel before commencing the treatment.

Most people adore having their feet worked on; indeed for many it is their favourite part of the body on which to receive a massage. Some, however, find it ticklish and uncomfortable. If this is the case, work firmly and apply more pressure to try to overcome the sensitivity. If this does not help, then it is usually best not to continue but to try again another day. In general, though, you can expect your massage in this area to be well received.

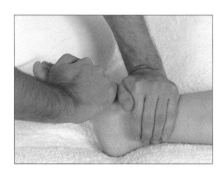

1 Kneel at the base of your partner's feet. Apply oil to your hands and gently make contact with your hands cupped around the foot and ankle, fingers pointing in opposite directions (*see above*). Avoid pulling the foot or applying any pressure at this point. Breathe in, and as you breathe out, glide your hands up sideways over the foot and onto the lower leg. When you reach the leg, turn your hands around to pull back towards yourself, gliding your upper hand underneath the foot and turning your lower one on to the foot (*see right*). As you pull your hands back towards you, lean back slightly to give the movement impact. Repeat this action three times.

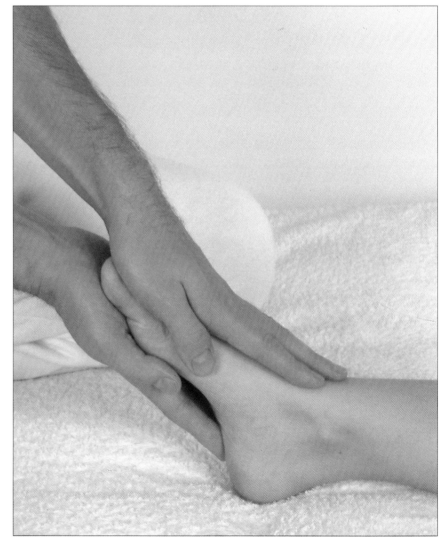

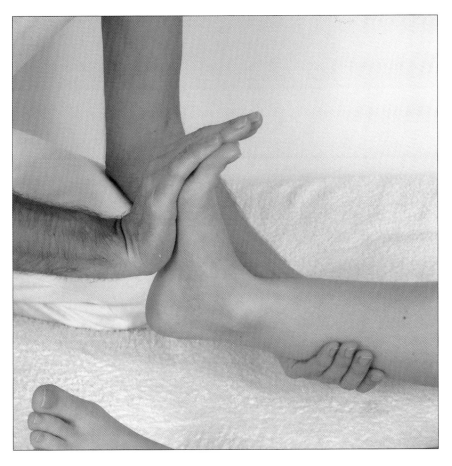

2 Place one hand flat on the sole of the foot, with the heel of your hand fitting securely into the instep. Hold the ankle firmly with your other hand. Breathe in, and as you breathe out, lean forward to push your hand gradually into the foot, towards your partner's knee. Hold the stretch for 10 seconds and repeat.

3 Place one hand on top of the leg, just above the ankle and wrap your other hand securely around the top of the foot. Breathe in, and as you breathe out, lean into the hand on the foot to gradually stretch the foot downwards. Be careful to apply the stretch very gradually and ask your partner to tell you when you have reached a comfortable point. Repeat once.

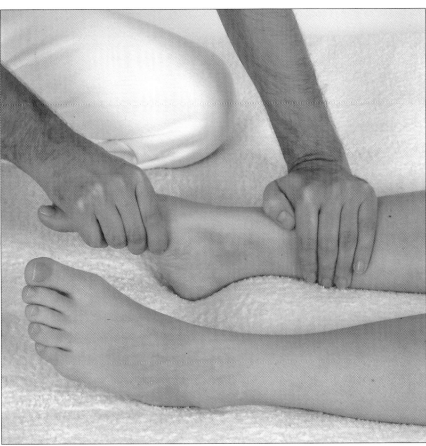

4 Wrap your hands around the sides of the foot, leaving the heels of your hands resting next to each other on top. You will need to be upright, over the foot, with straight arms to achieve this position. Lean into the heels of your hands to glide them firmly across the foot in opposite directions towards the fingers (*see right*). Continue the movement until you have covered the whole foot.

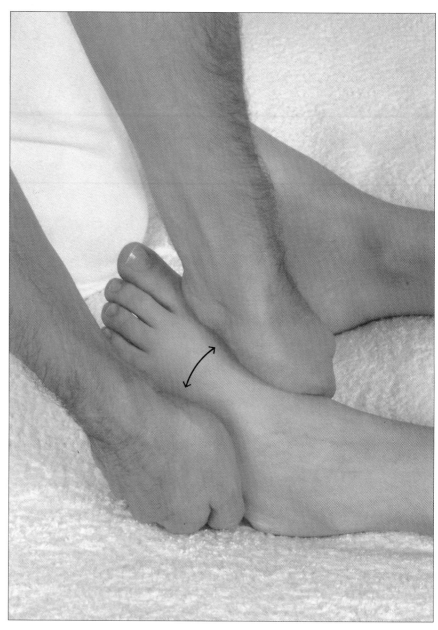

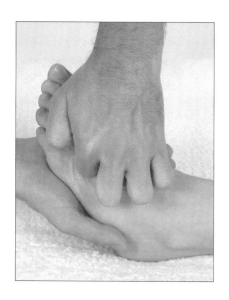

5 Hold the base of the foot firmly in one hand. Make your other hand into a fist and place it on the top of the foot. Rotate your fingers around to make small circular movements with your knuckles (*see above*). Work slowly and thoroughly all over the top of the foot, and carry out this movement three times.

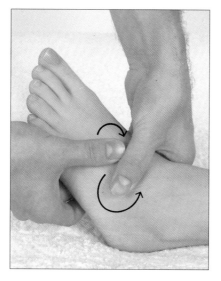

6 Wrap both hands around the foot leaving your thumbs free on the top (*see left*). Lean your thumbs in and slowly rotate them in small circles. Work evenly over the top of the foot and around the ankle-bone itself. Keep your thumbs straight and relaxed. Cover the entire foot in this way three times.

7 Hold the heel of the foot firmly with one hand and wrap the other hand around the top of the foot to leave your thumb on the sole of the foot. Press your thumb into the foot and slowly rotate in a small circle. Repeat until you have thoroughly covered the entire sole of the foot.

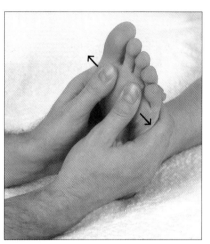

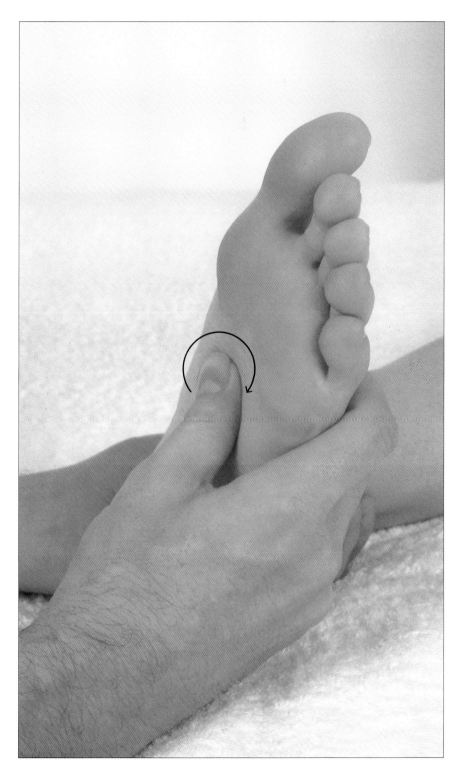

8 Wrap both hands around the front of the foot to leave thumbs free to work on the sole (*see above*). Make sure both thumbs are next to each other to begin the movement. Breathe in, and as you breathe out, lean into the tops of your thumbs to glide firmly across the foot in opposite directions. Extend the stroke right out to the edges of the foot. Repeat the movement until you have covered the entire foot. You may find that placing a pillow under your partner's foot makes this and the next movement more comfortable for you.

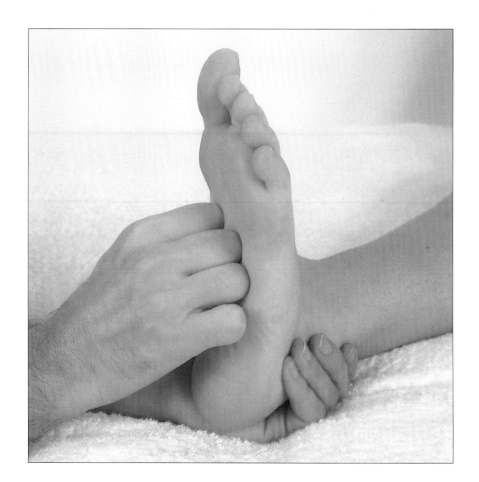

9 Hold the foot securely around the ankle with one hand. Make your other hand into a fist to knuckle over the sole of the foot, exactly as you did on the top of the foot. Rotate your fingers slowly over the entire sole of the foot, continuing around the ankle and the sides of the foot. Aim to cover the sole twice.

10 Hold the foot with one hand. Clasp the sides of the big toe between your finger and thumb and squeeze firmly. Pull the toe gently as your finger and thumb move up and off. If your partner finds this ticklish then it helps to be firmer and more assertive in your touch. Repeat the squeeze and pull with each of the toes, making sure to begin at the webs of the toes and to squeeze the sides rather than the top and bottom of each toe.

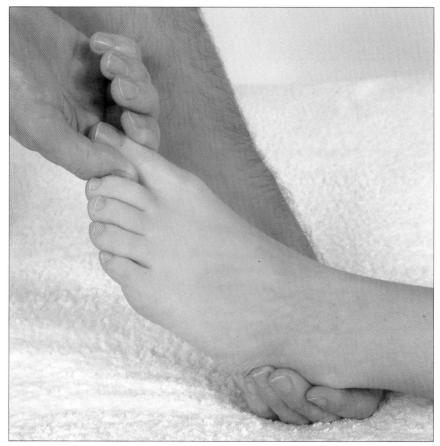

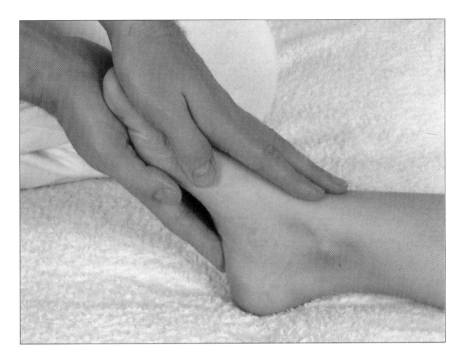

11 The stroke to complete this series is the effleurage that opened it. Wrap your hands around the foot, fingers pointing in opposite directions. Glide your hands over the foot up onto the lower leg. Turn the hands around to glide one hand underneath the foot and the other on top. Repeat the stroke three times and on the final stroke, maintain contact and hold the foot for 30 seconds to 'ground' your partner.

Common Ailments

Before you start to massage your partner, always ask if there are any physical problems. The following is a list of the most common complaints you are likely to come across when working on the front of the legs. It tells you what the best course of action is in each case: whether to massage or not and when medical attention is advisable.

● **Chilblains**
This is the ultimate symptom of poor circulation, and is exacerbated by a cold winter. Massage helps to stimulate, strengthen and invigorate the circulation, so encourage your partner to receive regular treatments. Marjoram or rosemary oils are stimulating, while camomile and lavender help to reduce the inflammation.

● **High Arch**
This results in a tense foot, which throws the balance out. It also encourages a person to clench the toes and generally overuse the muscles. Use massage and relaxing oils such as lavender and neroli to relax the tension.

● **Oedema**
This is most commonly known as 'water on the knee', and is characterized by inflammation and swelling within the joint capsule. It is caused by rheumatic or arthritic conditions, general wear and tear, a trauma such as an abrupt twist, or by synovitis, an inflammation of the synovial membranes. Massage with essential oils of lavender, camomile or juniper is useful in this case.

● **Strains and Sprains**
These involve tears to the muscle. A sprained ankle can be helped immediately by massage to reduce the swelling, to increase the circulation and to maintain the normal functioning of the leg muscles. A few days later you can work more around the immediate area. Months or even years later, you can work vigorously to soften any remaining scar tissue. Camomile and lavender oils will both help with the inflammation while marjoram, juniper and rosemary can be used later to invigorate and stimulate.

● **Swollen Ankles**
Trauma such as a kick, an insect bite, standing or sitting for long periods, or pre-menstrual tension can all result in swollen ankles. This is also a very common condition during pregnancy, when inactivity and the pressure of the foetus pressing on the pelvic veins makes it more difficult for the blood to return back up to the heart. It is also quite common among the elderly, especially if they take little exercise, as the heart will not pump so effectively. In all these circumstances, massage is extremely useful in helping the flow of circulation back up the legs to the heart. Light effleurage, concentrating on the area from the foot to the knee is the most useful, particularly if you continue for at least 30 strokes. Include the rest of the front-of-legs sequence if possible, but each time you effleurage repeat it at least 30 times. Juniper is an excellent oil to use for this type of water retention, but if your partner is pregnant, substitute lavender, rose or neroli.

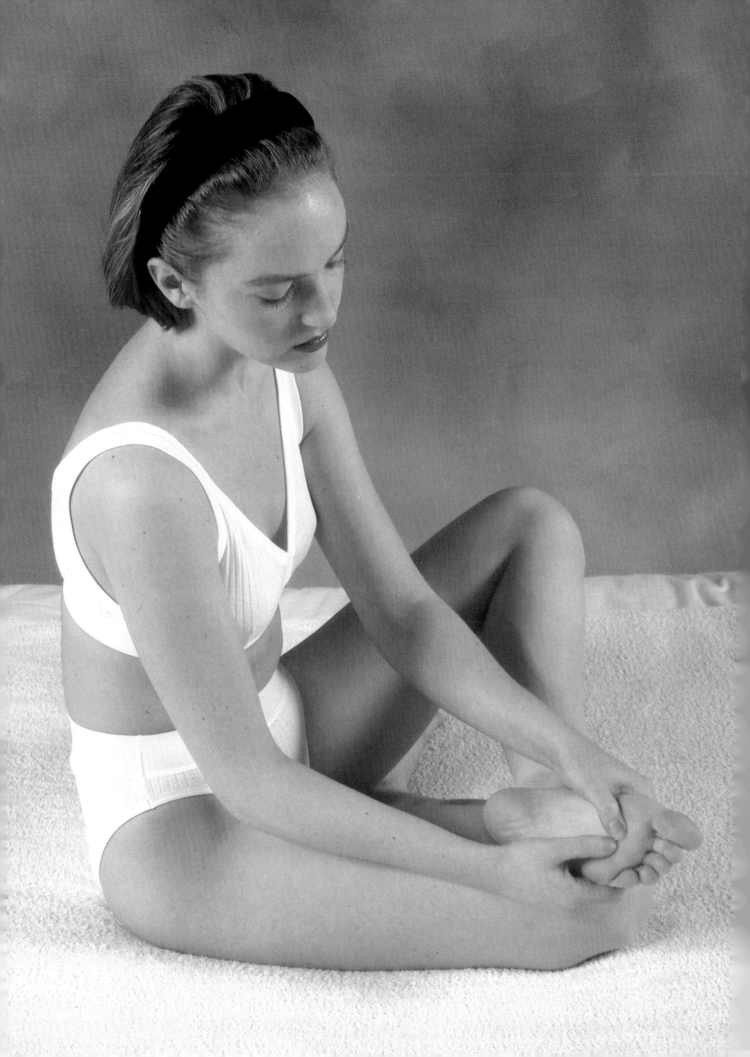

9

Self-Massage

Self-massage is one of the most loving and luxurious treats you can ever give yourself. It means lavishing time, care and attention on just you, taking responsibility for your own health and happiness, and treating yourself as your own best friend.

There can be no denying the unique experience of receiving massage from a caring friend or practitioner. Self-massage could never replace this, but it carries with it instead its own unique rewards. The most powerful of these is building a healthy, loving relationship with our own bodies. A recent survey in *New Woman* magazine revealed that only one woman in ten is happy with her body, and it is becoming clear that increasingly this problem is affecting men as well. The same survey revealed that women consistently use this as an excuse for not reaching out for what they really want in their lives. Feeling bad about our bodies inhibits our enjoyment of life – it is a human tragedy on a colossal scale.

To break out of this paralyzing cycle, we must accept and love ourselves as we are. We can always strive to improve our health and levels of fitness, but such striving is only healthy if we accept ourselves as fundamentally lovable and attractive, whatever improvements we feel we can make.

Massaging our bodies with love is the best way I know of generating more respect for ourselves. It is only when we feel respect, peace and happiness within that life can be fun, light-hearted and enjoyable, and it is only when we accept and care for ourselves that we can accept and care for others.

Massaging your own body is the
best way of showing love for yourself. You
can luxuriate in exotic oils or choose a
sequence or two to refresh yourself
at any time of day.

Self-Massage Without Oil

The following self-massage sequence is wonderfully versatile and can be carried out almost anywhere. Oil is not necessary and you do not have to remove any clothing. All you need is a table to rest your arms on, though you could still carry out many of the movements in the sequence without one.

You could spend from 5 to 20 minutes working with the sequence. Even 5 minutes will make a difference and you can use some movements, such as the pressure on the eyes, to great effect by themselves. This particular stroke is a very old yoga movement. It helps to relax and strengthen the eye muscles, reduce eye-strain and improve the eyesight.

Make a conscious effort to let go of your head and neck as you perform the movements. Allow the weight to create pressure effortlessly so you do not have to press your hands or fingers accurately into any areas to create a dynamic.

Releasing pressure from your face, neck and shoulders like this on a regular basis is one of the best guarantees you can have against a prematurely aged appearance.

1 Lean your face into your hand, eyes resting into the heels of your hands, fingers anchored on your forehead (*see right*). Make sure you are sitting close enough to the table to let your arms and the rest of your body relax completely. Hold the position for at least 30 seconds.

2 Bring the heels of your hands onto your eyebrows. Breathe in, and as you breathe out, glide your hands slowly across the eyebrows onto the temples to the ears (*see below*). Continue this movement across the forehead until you have covered it right up to the hairline.

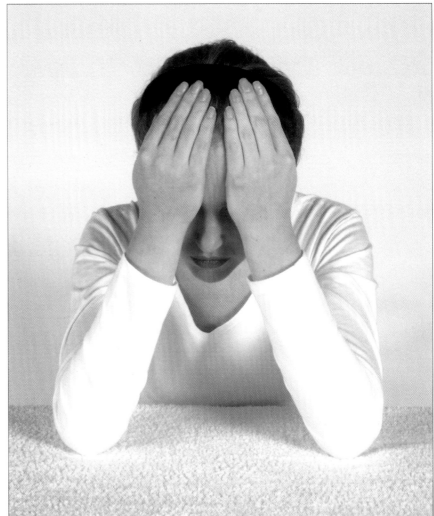

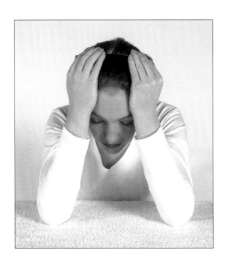

3 Bring your middle two fingers to rest on your temples. Let your neck and head release as much as possible to be supported by the pressure of your fingers. Breathe in, and as you breathe out, slowly rotate your fingers in a clockwise direction at least five times (*see right*). To add variety to this stroke, simply maintain a stationary pressure here without rotating your fingers. This is particularly useful if you have a headache coming from a dull ache in the temples.

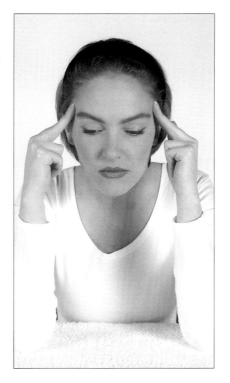

4 Place the ball of your thumbs just underneath the inner edge of your eyebrows (*see below*). This can be quite a tender area so you may need to control the pressure you apply here and inhibit the entire weight of your head. Follow your instincts: use the amount of pressure you feel comfortable with. Hold the pressure for 10 seconds; release and hold for another 10 seconds. This is a very useful point to massage if you are suffering from tired eyes, headaches or sinus congestion.

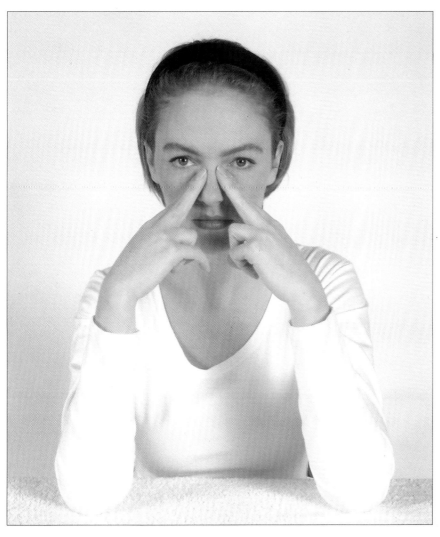

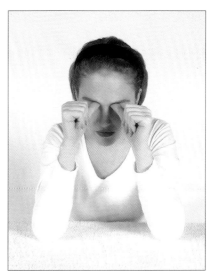

5 Place your middle two fingers either side of the nose at the top. Breathe in, and as you breathe out, slowly glide the fingers down the nose, over the nostrils and onto the cheeks (*see left*). Do this just once, unless you are suffering from sinusitis, in which case it will help to repeat five times.

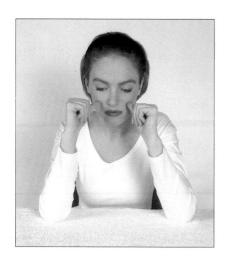

6 Place the balls of your thumbs under your cheek-bones, just either side of the nostrils, resting the weight of your head and neck into your thumbs. Breathe in, and as you breathe out, slowly glide your thumbs across the cheek-bones and up to the ears (*see above*). You can also use your thumbs to maintain stationary pressure, holding the point for 10 seconds, then repeating further along until you have reached the ears. This is good for sinus congestion.

7 Take hold of your jawbone at the point of the chin, between your fingers and thumb. Press firmly into the jaw. Breathe in, and as you breathe out, slowly rotate your fingers into the bone, keeping your thumbs pressed firmly in at the same time. Work outwards up to the ears on either side (*see right*). Repeat five times if you suffer from jaw-tension or grind your teeth at night.

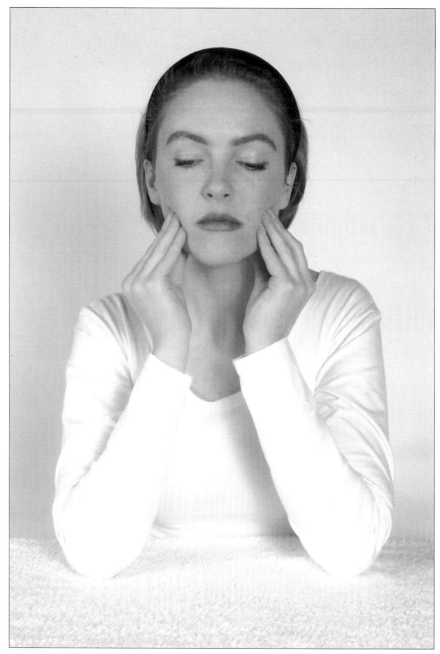

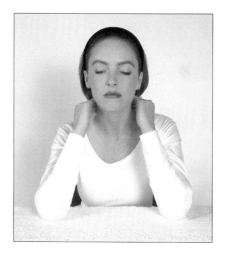

8 Place your fingers on the top of the neck behind the ears. Lean your head forward slightly so that you stretch the muscles and make them more accessible. Breathe in, and as you breathe out, lean the pads of your fingers into either side of the neck and rotate slowly. Make sure that you keep pressing your fingers into the neck as you rotate them. Work slowly and thoroughly down to the base of the neck (*see left*). Repeat this movement at least twice if your neck is stiff or you have a headache due to neck-tension.

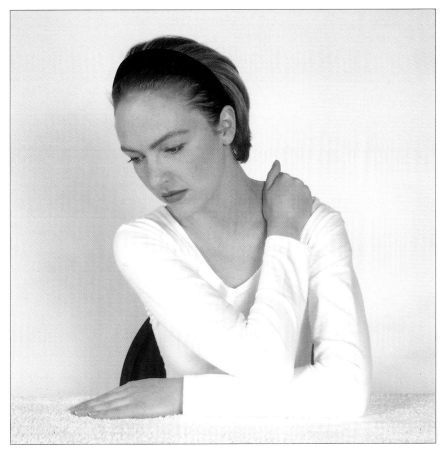

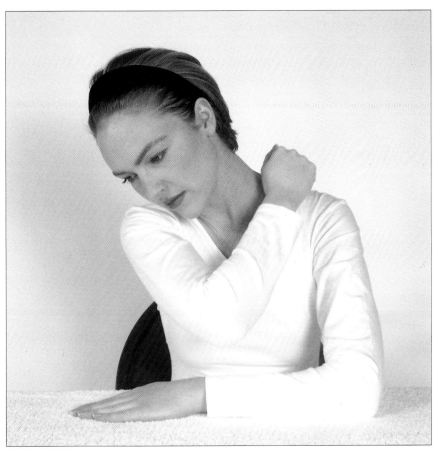

9 Rest one hand on the table and bring your other hand to work on the opposite shoulder (*see left*). Begin nearest the neck, tilting your head slightly to one side to make it easier to work here. Squeeze the muscle slowly and deeply between the heel of your hand and your fingers. Continue this movement along the length of the muscle to your shoulder joint. Repeat twice.

10 Place the pads of your fingers on top of the shoulder muscle, beginning nearest the neck. Breathe in, and as you breathe out, press your fingers into the muscle and rotate slowly. Move along the top of the muscle in this way (*see below*). Check that you are still pressing your fingers into the muscle as you rotate them, or you will work too lightly to have an effect. Repeat twice.

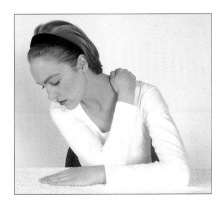

11 Bring your hand up to your shoulder. Make it into a relaxed fist shape. Breathe in, and as you breathe out, bounce your fist up and down on the side of your neck and shoulder (*see left*). Begin lightly and gently, gradually increasing the impact. Make the movement rapid, keeping your fist close to your neck and shoulder. Keep breathing as you work to release and let go of the tightness. This is a very powerful way to free up chronic tension in this area. Repeat movements 9, 10 and 11 on the other side of the body.

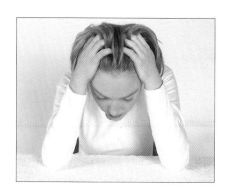

12 Rest your elbows on the table again. Place the heels of your hands just behind the hairline (*see left*). Release the weight of your head and neck. Breathe in, and as you breathe out, slowly rotate the heels of your hands, keeping the pressure firm. Work thoroughly over the front and the sides of your head and as much of the back as you can comfortably reach.

13 Slide your fingers into your hair and draw your hands through it from the roots to the ends (*see below*). Work thoroughly, one hand after the other, to cover both the front and the back of the head. This is a very easy stroke to carry out. It should feel very easy and pleasant, and together with the previous stroke, will help to alleviate headaches at the front of the head.

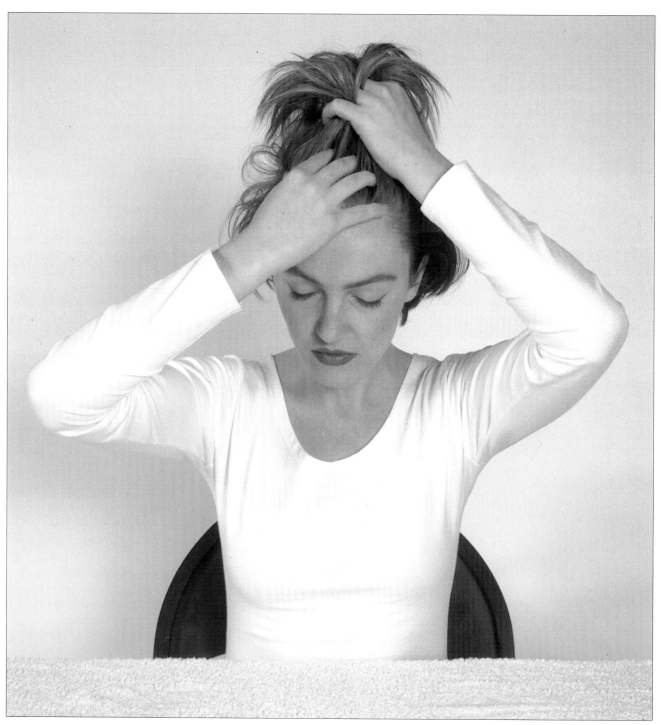

Self-Massage
With Oil

This routine is simple, straightforward and wonderfully luxurious. It is an opportunity to really indulge yourself with your favourite oils and creams. You can either pick and choose specific strokes, complete the entire sequence in 10 minutes or be really generous and spend a whole hour over it. There can be few treats more refreshing than soaking in a luxurious scented bath, then massaging yourself with a creamy lotion or nourishing oil.

You do not get the profound relaxation that comes from receiving a treatment from someone else, but working on yourself has its benefits. The deep kneading and pummelling work on the thighs (*see steps 11, 12, and 13, page 151 and step 14, page 152*) really gets your circulation moving and a daily routine will help you rid yourself of any fluid retention or cellulite.

Choose the most comfortable position, either sitting in an armchair or on the floor. Make sure that you give yourself plenty of time to get familiar with the strokes when you first come to this routine. I can think of no better way to spend a quiet evening alone.

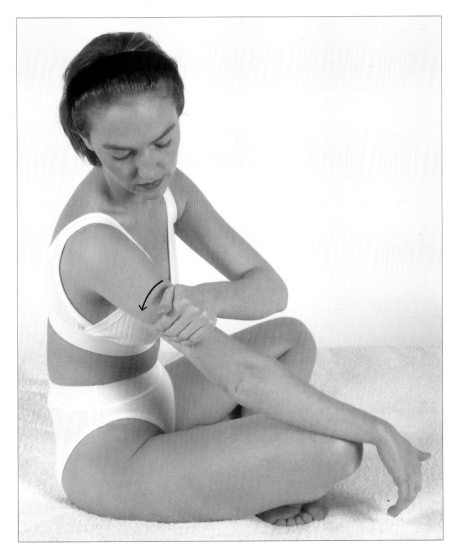

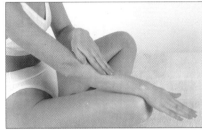

Arms and
Hands

1 Sit comfortably, supporting yourself in an easy chair if you like. Apply oil to your hand. Glide up the arm you are working on, smooth around the shoulder joint and down to your hand again (*see above*). Concentrate on the upward stroke to stimulate the flow of lymph and blood to the armpit. Repeat three times.

2 Wrap your hand around your upper arm. Squeeze the flesh and muscle between your fingers and the heel of your hand (*see left*). Begin at the top of the arm and squeeze along the outside down to your elbow. Then return to the top of the arm and repeat the movement on the front of your upper arm down to your elbow.

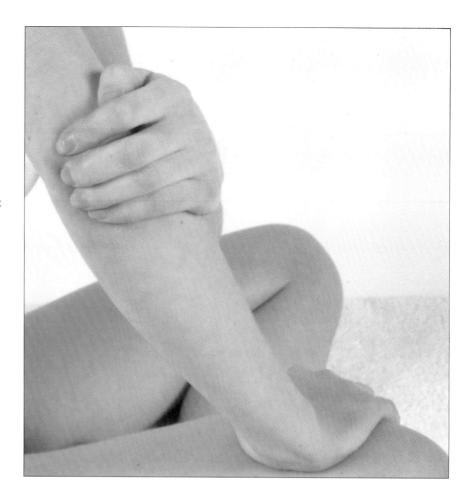

3 Wrap your hand around your elbow and place your fingers on the bone (*see right*). Use your fingers to rotate one large circle on the elbow. Then work into the grooves and indentations around the bone. Massage your fingers thoroughly into the entire joint and think of clearing out any congestion or waste products that may have collected here.

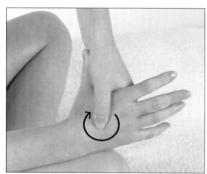

4 Hold your hand to work with your thumb on the back of your hand (*see above*). Breathe in, and as you breathe out, lean your thumb into the back of your hand. Rotate in small circles over the entire area.

5 Turn your hand over to work with your thumb on the palm. Lean your thumb in and rotate in small circles, moving over the entire area (*see right*). Concentrate on the thick pads of muscle at each side, which tend to store tension from everyday activities like driving and typing.

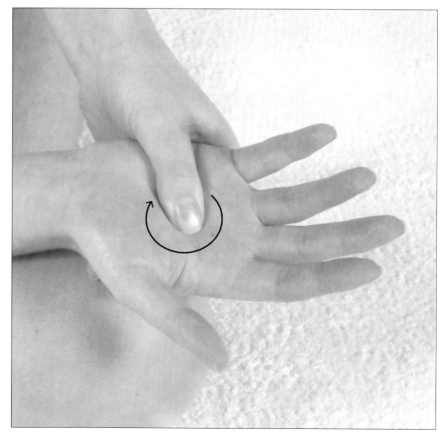

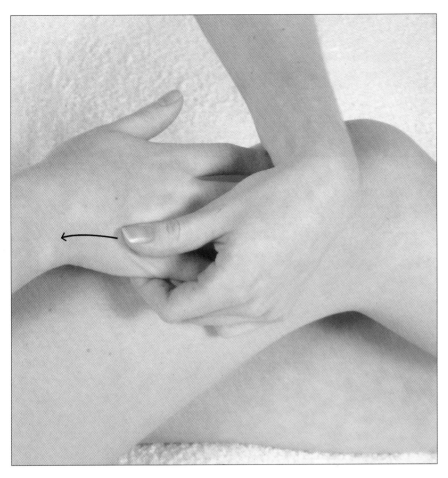

6 Glide your thumb between the tendons running down the back of your hand (*see left*). Work down from your fingers towards your wrist. Begin with the tendon running from your little finger and work down each one towards your thumb. In reflexology this is the zone that governs the lymphatic system.

7 Squeeze the sides of each finger between your finger and thumb (*see below*). Work from the base of the fingers down to the tip, squeezing as you move down each finger, pulling towards you. At the tip of the finger, squeeze and pull each one. Make sure that you squeeze thoroughly at the ends of your fingers; this area corresponds to the sinuses in reflexology.

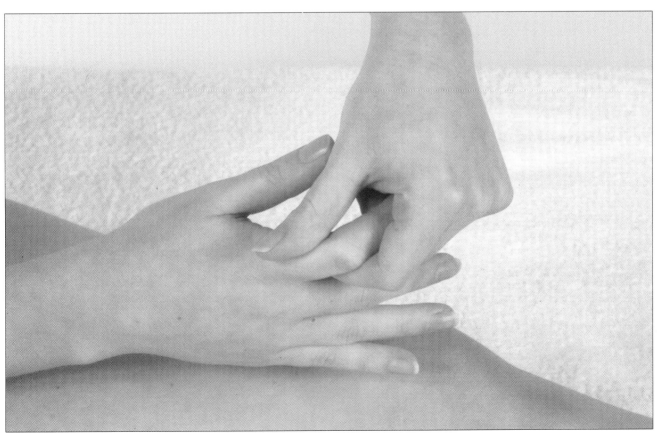

Chest and Abdomen

1 Bring your hand to the pectoral muscle just next to your armpit. Anchor your fingers into the armpit and squeeze the heel of your hand firmly into the muscle (*see right*). You will find it easier if you do not have clothes in your way. When you have worked thoroughly into the muscle, repeat the movement on your other side. Avoid using too much oil or your hand will slip off the skin.

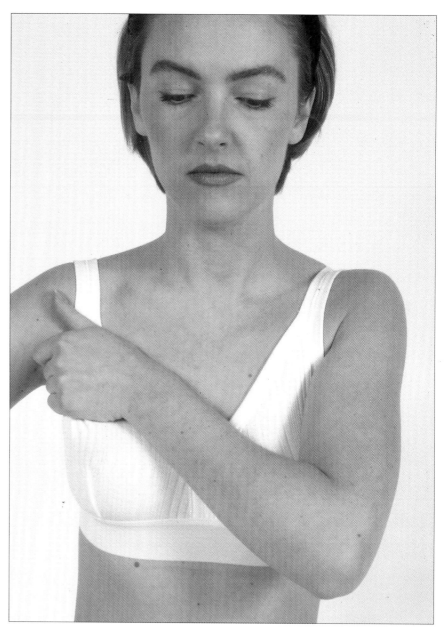

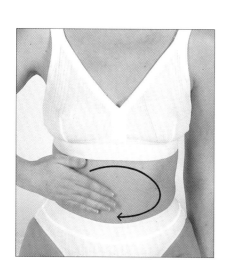

2 Bring one hand to your abdomen and circle it slowly in a clockwise direction (*see above*). Cover the entire abdomen from your ribcage down to the pubic bone adjusting the pressure to your own comfort. Again this is best done without clothes restricting the extent of your stroke. Use this stroke daily to help with both digestion and the movement of waste products through the colon.

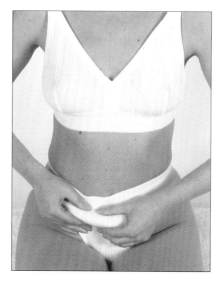

3 Bring both hands to your abdomen and pick up the flesh between your fingers and thumb (*see left*). Squeeze it and roll it to knead the flesh and muscles using as much pressure as you can comfortably tolerate. Work systematically over the whole abdomen. Use this stroke regularly if you suffer from water retention or abdominal bloating and you will soon feel the benefits.

Legs and Feet

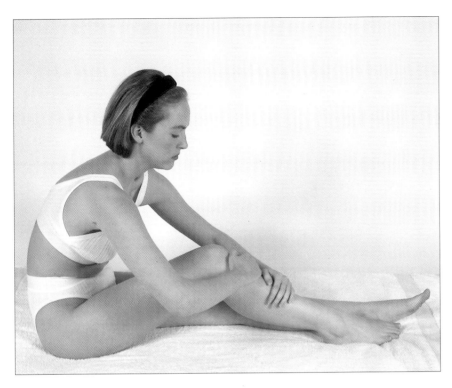

1 You may be most comfortable sitting in an armchair with your feet resting on your coffee table. Otherwise simply bend one leg up towards yourself (*see top left*). Glide your hands up from your foot over your calf and onto your thigh, at least five times. If you want to concentrate on your thighs, simply repeat the effleurage from your knee up to the top of your thigh.

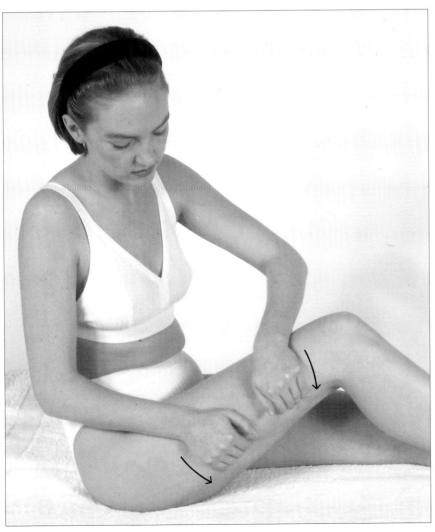

2 Bring your hands to your other thigh. Lean the heel of your hands into your thigh and squeeze firmly towards your fingers (*see bottom left*). Anchor your fingers firmly on the leg so they do not slip. This stroke is also excellent on the inside of your thighs. Simply turn your hands around, fingers pointing to the floor. Lean your heels in and squeeze towards your fingers.

3 Make your hands into a fist. Place your knuckles just above the knee. Breathe in, and as you breathe out, press into and glide up the thigh, one hand after the other (*see below*). Work thoroughly up the front of your thigh, then the outer and inner thigh. This stroke can be painful on the outer thigh if there is water retention or cellulite.

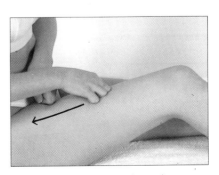

151

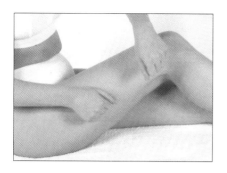

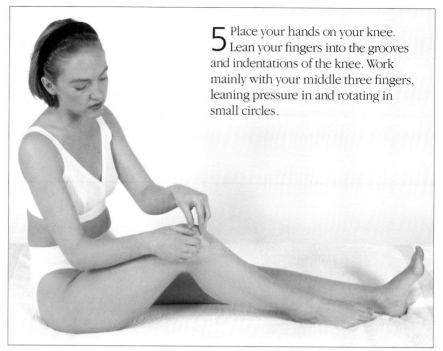

5 Place your hands on your knee. Lean your fingers into the grooves and indentations of the knee. Work mainly with your middle three fingers, leaning pressure in and rotating in small circles.

4 Keep your hands in the fist-like shape that you adopted in step 3. Place the flat part of your fist, between your knuckles and your finger-joints, on your thigh (*see above*). Bounce your fists lightly on your thigh, letting your hand spring away as it touches the skin. Work vigorously in this way up and down the thigh until you feel you have thoroughly covered the entire thigh.

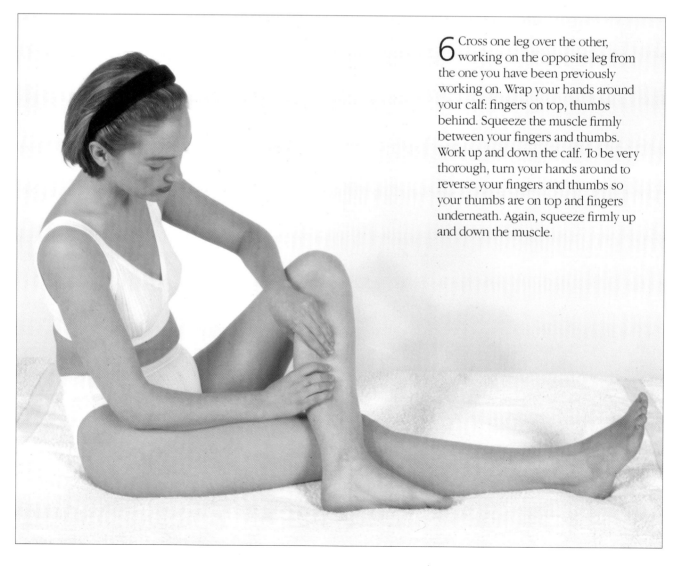

6 Cross one leg over the other, working on the opposite leg from the one you have been previously working on. Wrap your hands around your calf: fingers on top, thumbs behind. Squeeze the muscle firmly between your fingers and thumbs. Work up and down the calf. To be very thorough, turn your hands around to reverse your fingers and thumbs so your thumbs are on top and fingers underneath. Again, squeeze firmly up and down the muscle.

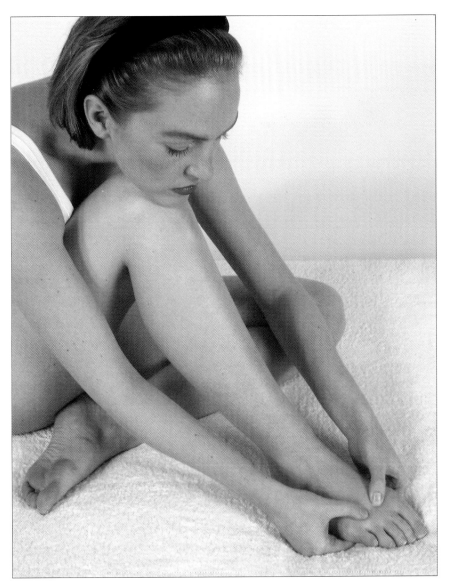

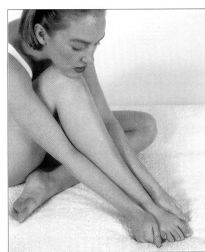

7 Lean over to reach your foot. Place the heels of your hands sideways on the foot, fingers wrapped underneath. Breathe in, and as you breathe out, glide your hands firmly across your foot (*see above*). Push your fingers up into your foot to stretch and expand the top of your foot. Repeat five times.

8 Bring your thumbs to the foot. Breathe in, and as you breathe out, lean your thumbs in and rotate in small circles over the top of your foot (*see left*). Pay attention to any painful areas. Return to them after you have covered the foot. A variation is to hold the foot with one hand and work with only one thumb.

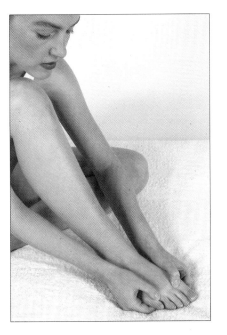

9 This stroke feels as though you are clearing between the tendons on your feet. Wrap your hands around the foot as before. Bring your thumbs to glide down the furrows running from the toes, between the tendons, up to the ankle (*see left*). Work with either both thumbs or one thumb at a time. According to reflexology this stimulates the lungs.

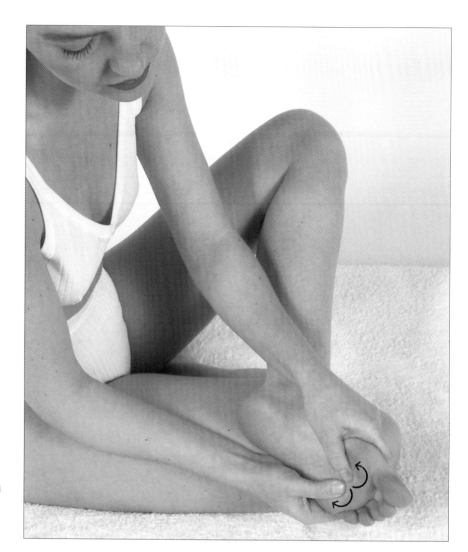

10 Bring your foot to rest on your knee so you can comfortably reach the side of your foot. Do not change feet – the pictures show the opposite foot for a clear view. Wrap your hands around the foot, leaving your thumbs to work on the sole. Lean in and rotate your thumbs in small circles. Continue until you have covered the entire sole.

11 Clasp your foot firmly in one hand, resting the foot on your inside thigh. Make your other hand into a fist, keeping your wrist relaxed, and gently pound it on the sole of your foot. Work carefully over the entire area, especially the heel, and extend out to the sides of your foot. Work close to the foot, letting your fist spring back each time you contact your foot. This is a very invigorating movement that prepares your foot for the next movement.

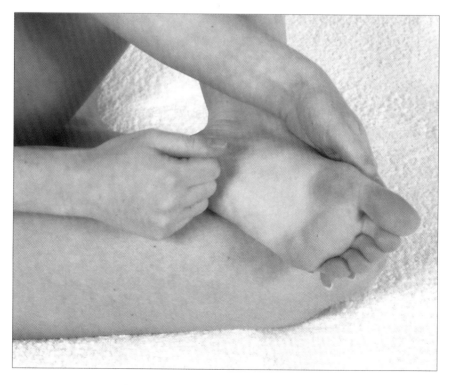

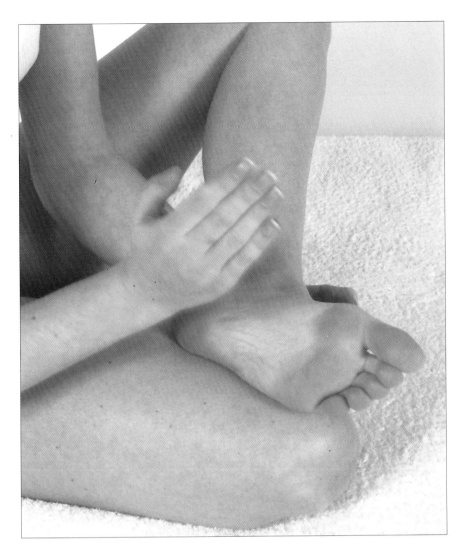

12 Keeping your foot in exactly the same position, hold your hand out straight and hit the sole of your foot with the side of your hand. Keep your hand close to the foot (*see left*). Check that your wrist and hand are relaxed. As you make contact on the foot each time, let the little finger bounce into the hand.

13 Enclose the sides of each toe between your forefinger and thumb. Squeeze gently, pull, stretch and twist them as you slide your fingers down and off the tip (*see below*). Use a firm tugging movement with each toe. Finish with a soothing stroke down the entire foot. Go back to step 1 and treat the other leg.

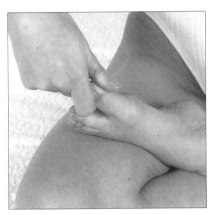

Common Ailments

Massaging yourself not only stimulates the circulation and leaves you feeling relaxed and invigorated, it also relieves a number of ailments.

● **Abdominal Bloatedness**
Effleurage and kneading on the abdomen will help (see steps 2 and 3, page 150). Do this every day, first thing in the morning and again in the evening. A combination of juniper, geranium and rosemary essential oils is very effective.

● **Digestive Upset**
Apply slow effleurage to the abdomen (see step 2, page 150). Use a combination of peppermint and lavender oils.

● **Eye strain**
For headaches caused by eyestrain and for blurred vision with a migraine, lean your palms into your eyes (see step 1, page 142). After 20 seconds of pressure, rotate the heels of your hands slowly in large circles in the eye sockets.

● **Tired Feet**
Even a short massage can help enormously. According to reflexology, you will also be toning up the entire body as you contact the reflex points of each organ, gland and structure in the body. Structural problems such as a high or fallen arch will also improve significantly. For a fallen arch,

work vigorously to tone and stimulate the foot. With a high arch, work slowly to relax the foot.

● **Varicose Veins**
Light effleurage strokes up the legs will help poor circulation. Raise your legs to take off the pressure and to ease the upward flow of blood and fluid. Avoid working directly on top of the veins if they are very pronounced and painful. Keep the kneading movements for your thighs. If you have broken capillaries here, avoid the pummelling stroke (see step 14, page 152), knuckling (see step 13, page 151) and vigorous kneading, as they could make them worse.

Which Way Now?

Happiness is feeling good about yourself.
LOUISE HAY

Congratulations! You are now well on your way to mastering a uniquely therapeutic and life-enhancing skill. By now you will have had the opportunity to practise some, if not all, of the routines in the book. You will, most likely, have received enthusiastic responses from those that you have worked on and, hopefully, you will have experienced some massage on yourself.

It is a good idea to receive massage as you learn, so that you know the experience first hand. Then you can understand how just a simple effleurage stroke can soothe and renew, how music played just a fraction too loud can disturb or how a chilly room can ruin the entire treatment. If you share this book with a partner, you can both develop and fine tune your approach. Receiving and enjoying the benefits of massage will also leave you feeling inspired and motivated to practise. It is also important to take care of yourself when you are giving to others in this way, or you may find yourself feeling deplete, and wishing you were on the receiving end. If you ever feel this, simply get a massage yourself. Ideally you should only ever massage when you really want to and are feeling well – it is unfair to both you and your partner to give a massage if you are feeling ambivalent about it or physically below par.

The right approach
When giving massage your attitude is of paramount importance. To give a worthwhile treatment, you need to free yourself of preoccupations and physical tension. Use the guidelines outlined in 'Preparation' (*see pages 12–15*) for a simple relaxation routine. Essentially you need to be calm and focused when you massage, letting your thoughts pass by as they come to you, until you are in a state of relaxed alertness, with your intuition heightened. If you feel drawn

to concentrate on a particular area of your partner's body, trust yourself.

Your intuition will also help you to sense how people are feeling. When they come for a treatment, make a note of your first impression of them, and think of a quality you would like to instil in them through your massage. If you feel they look drained and dejected, and you decide to inject energy and confidence through your hands, you may be surprised to see the difference this makes. As you kneel alongside them, before or during making contact, visualize a ball of white light above your head, see the light as containing the positive qualities you wish your partner to receive. As you breathe in, see the light pouring in through you to your arms and hands, then carry on with your treatment, trusting that the quality of your touch will convey your intention to your partner.

Adding variety to your treatments
When you are fully competent at all the strokes and routines, you may notice yourself getting bored. This happens to massage therapists who have been taught a rigid format which allows no scope for their intuition or creativity to come into play.

Every treatment you give needs to be different and unique. Even if you massage the same person week after week, their needs are never exactly the same. Approach every treatment, however long or short, with a fresh outlook and check how your partner is feeling on that particular occasion. Some people have a clear idea of how they would like to feel at the end of the treatment, which areas need more attention and where they would like you to begin the treatment. If it feels appropriate, vary your routine by starting work on the front of the body. If your partner has been coming to you regularly, monitor progress – the changes you see will act as a great spur to you. Allow yourself to work intuitively on the problem areas, make up your own strokes or adapt them from other routines and work with your eyes closed to enhance the sensitivity of your hands. The greatest massage practitioners in the Orient have traditionally been the blind who have to rely on their hands to see the world around them.

Take into account the time of day you carry out a treatment and find out what your partner is doing afterwards. If it is a morning session or your partner is on the way to work, avoid too relaxing a treatment. To offer a more stimulating massage, work faster and more vigorously in all your movements, including the effleurage. Keep your strokes steady and rhythmic and avoid any jerkiness as you speed up. My recommendation is that you begin on the head and face so your partner benefits from the profound relaxation working this brings. Continue working on the front of the body at your normal pace. Then, when your friend turns over, work on the back, increasing the speed of your strokes. Finish by working on the legs, with strong and vigorous effleurage strokes. Include the percussion strokes – pummelling and hacking – and finish by hacking on the soles of the feet. After that, your partner should be ready to run a marathon or simply to handle a busy day at work.

Keeping fit and healthy

Giving massage, especially a vigorous, stimulating one, can be demanding. Your own health and level of fitness needs to be good, so you are not exhausted or drained by the exertion. You may want to review your state of health by checking that your diet is supporting you. If in doubt, see a nutritionist or dietary therapist – the more you investigate and experiment with the complementary therapies, the more your knowledge will help other people. Receiving massage is often the first step for people to explore and enhance their health. If they are chronically fatigued or suffer from persistent premenstrual tension, they may welcome further recommendations from you about other therapies. The more you take responsibility for enhancing your own well-being and make use of

homoeopathy, acupuncture, herbalism and all the holistic approaches, the more you will be a living example of good health.

The most common complaint I hear from new students is how their legs ache after giving a treatment on the floor. This is understandable if your muscles are simply not used to kneeling for long periods of time. However, it also indicates that you are not as supple as you might be. Attend a good yoga or stretch class in your area at least twice a week and begin to include a daily stretching session at home when you are relaxing in the evening, even in front of the television. The more comfortable and relaxed you are while you give massage and the more you focus on the treatment, the more you and your partner will enjoy the treatment. Massage will be no joy if you are in agony.

Similarly you will find massage a strain if you are overweight. You are likely to perspire and feel uncomfortable and may need to limit the length of the treatment to 30 minutes. If you feel you need to postpone giving massage until you are healthier yourself, make sure you receive plenty of treatments yourself, eat good quality food and apply yourself to an exercise programme. Feeling good about yourself is the best incentive for reducing weight, increasing your health and enhancing the quality of your life.

By now you will realize that giving good quality massage depends a great deal on your own vitality and well-being. Students who are committed to improving the quality of their energy, frequently embark on personal growth pursuits for themselves. It is not unusual for people to experience big changes in their own lives as they become involved in massage. I frequently see students change the entire structure of their lives during a course – as they get more in touch with themselves, they become less tolerant of relationships or jobs that are not fulfilling. Within the safe setting of the massage class, problems can be aired and support given. Advanced students are encouraged to look at themselves in depth and to work on their own emotional, physical and spiritual health. The more harmony and balance you have in your life, the more equipped you are to give quality time, attention and care to others.

Your prime intention in giving massage is to instil a sense of calm – an elusive quality in the normal hubbub of daily life. Since you must be able to experience stillness in yourself before you can pass this on to others, you may want to explore approaches such as meditation, yoga and Tai-Chi, and find one that suits you. Personally I have studied and applied each of these at different stages of my life, and all have contributed enormously to my own peace and contentment.

Tai-Chi is a form of moving meditation developed in China generations ago. It consists of a series of slow dance-like movements which still the mind, relax the body and focus your awareness on moving from the centre of your body. It also strengthens and enhances your own vitality, leaving you feeling more grounded and at ease with your own body. I noticed all these benefits after my first class. Find a good teacher and try it for yourself.

Spreading the joy of massage
I hope this book gives you as much pleasure and satisfaction as I have experienced during my years of practise and teaching. I have been privileged to witness the joy people derive from giving to others through massage – it is an instinctive and natural desire in all of us. I have seen 'strangers' feel more at ease with each other after a few weeks of exchanging massage than with friends they have known for years. Massage is one of the most positive, life-affirming practices we possess.

Massage utterly changed my life. It brought me down to earth and directly into contact with my own buried conflicts. It sent me on a voyage of self-discovery and opened up a new world for me. Understandably, I am totally committed to spreading the power of massage to everyone.

I believe massage should be a part of our everyday life that we share with friends and family. It would transform the quality of communication within families, and reduce the manic anxiety that consumes so much of our day-to-day life. If each of us creates a pocket of peace inside us, it spreads to the people around us, so adding a little each time to the health of the entire planet.

Further Reading

Chaitow, Leon. *Vaccination & Immunization – Dangers, Delusions & Alternatives*, Saffron Walden, C.W. Daniel, 1987

Chopra, Dr Deepak. *Perfect Health*, New York, Bantam Books, 1992

Chopra, Dr Deepak. *Unconditional Life*, New York, Bantam Books, 1991

Curtis, Susan and Fraser, Romy. *Natural Healing for Women*, London, Pandora Press, 1991

Dawes, Nigel and Harrold, Fiona. *Massage Cures*, Wellingborough, Thorsons, 1990

Downing, George. *The Massage Book*, London, Arkana, 1989

Dychtwald, Ken. *Bodymind*, Los Angeles, Jeremy P. Tarcher, 1977

Hay, Louise. *You Can Heal Your Life*, London, Eden Grove Editions, 1988

Juhan, Deane. *Job's Body*, New York, Station Hill Press, 1987

Kurtz, Ron and Prestera, Dr Hector. *The Body Reveals*, New York, Harper & Row, 1970

Lidell, Lucinda *et al*. *The Book of Massage*, London, Ebury Press, 1984

Liechti, Elaine. *Shiatsu – Japanese Massage for Health and Fitness*, Shaftesbury, Element Books, 1992

Manning, Matthew. *The Power is Within You: Matthew Manning's Guide to Self-healing*, Wellingborough, Thorsons, 1991

Miller, Alice. *Breaking Down the Wall of Silence*, London, Virago, 1992

Montagu, Ashley. *Touching – The Human Significance of the Skin*, New York, Harper & Row, 1970

Proto, Louis. *Self-healing – Use Your Mind to Heal Your Body*, London, Piatkus Books, 1990

Ryman, Daniele. *The Aromatherapy Handbook*, Saffron Walden, C.W. Daniel, 1989

Siegal, Dr Bernie S. *Love, Medicine & Miracles*, London, Arrow Books, 1991

Wawood, Valerie Ann. *The Fragrant Pharmacy*, London, Bantam, 1991

Wilson, Kathleen J.W. *Anatomy & Physiology in Health & Illness*, Edinburgh, Churchill Livingstone, 1963

Young, Jacqueline. *Vital Energy*, London/Sevenoaks, Headway, 1991.

Index

Acknowledgements

I would like to thank my teachers who have, over the past ten years, inspired me and enriched the quality of my life immeasurably. Fiona Shaw, my early mentor and guide; Brygette Ryley and Gabrielle Gad, who taught me to connect body and mind, and Carola Beresford-Cooke for her wonderful Shiatsu teaching.

My students who have, over the years, constantly reinspired me and reaffirmed the power of massage for me. Their enthusiasm has never allowed me to become blasé as I have watched so many people benefit enormously.

All the people behind the scenes who contributed to making this book so beautiful. Everyone at Eddison Sadd Editions: Hilary Krag and Elaine Partington for their flair and hard work on the design; Michele Doyle for supporting me and editing so thoroughly and discreetly, and Ian Jackson for seeing the potential of the book in the first place. Sue Atkinson for her exquisite and precise photography; Alastair Greetham for his advice and input; Alastair Frazer and Carol Knight for their prompt and efficient typing. Finally, my wonderful models who were forever patient and enthusiastic: Marc Salnicki, Nicole Bainbridge and Debbie Mason. It is a great tribute to the powerful appeal of touch that everyone involved in the making of this book eventually enrolled on a course at the London College of Massage and embraced massage into their lives.

All the teachers and staff at the London College of Massage who have supported me tremendously throughout the writing of this book: Isabelle Hughes, Patsy Batchelor, Alex Mavolwane, Marc Salnicki, Audrey Choules, Debbie Mellor, John White and Fiona McGregor.

Finally, I want to thank my son Jamie for putting up with me being so preoccupied, and Charlotte for helping us through.

Fiona Harrold

For massage courses and treatments contact
The London College of Massage:

5–6 Newman Passage, London W1P 3PF.
Telephone 0171–323 3574

1 Lansdowne Terrace, Patrick's Hill, Cork, Ireland.
Telephone (010353) 21 500509

Art Director Elaine Partington
Art Editor Hilary Krag
Editor Michele Doyle
Copy-editor Rosanne Hooper
Proof-readers Zoë Hughes and William Gleeson
Production Hazel Kirkman and Charles James
Indexer Dorothy Frame
Illustrator Gordon Munro
Photographer Sue Atkinson
Consultant Physiotherapist Alastair Greetham

Clothing courtesy of Million Dollar Sports and Strip at Garage,
King's Road, London SW3.
Futon supplied by Futon Company;
169 Tottenham Court Road, London W1P 9LH.
Telephone 0171-636 9984